NURSING ETHICS FOR MODERN HEALTHCARE

NURSING ETHICS FOR MODERN HEALTHCARE

ALLISON J. TERRY

cognella
SAN DIEGO

Bassim Hamadeh, CEO and Publisher
Amanda Martin, Executive Publisher
Alverne Ball, Project Editor
Jeanine Rees, Production Editor
Jess Estrella, Senior Graphic Designer
Laura Duncan, Licensing Specialist
Natalie Piccotti, Director of Marketing
Kassie Graves, Senior Vice President, Editorial
Alia Bales, Director, Project Editorial and Production

Printed in the United States of America.

cognella® | ACADEMIC PUBLISHING
320 South Cedros Ave., Ste. 400, Solana Beach, CA 92075

BRIEF CONTENTS

DETAILED CONTENTS

CHAPTER 1

INTRODUCTION TO ETHICS

CHAPTER OBJECTIVES

After studying this chapter, students will be able to:

- Discuss the difference in ethics, values, and morals.
- Describe the National League for Nursing's core values that are intrinsic to nursing education.
- Discuss the differences between the deontological view and the consequential view of various ethical issues.
- Analyze the difference between moral reflection and ethical competence.
- Discuss the various provisions of the Code of Ethics of the American Nurses' Association.

KEY TERMS

bioethics
Code of Ethics for Nurses With Interpretive Statements
consequentialism
deontology
ethical competence
ethics
moral reflection
morals
Nightingale pledge
utilitarianism
values

Few would dispute the necessity of nurses having a clear understanding of ethics, values, and morals, as well as the ability to recognize when nursing care is being implemented in an ethical manner. The recent pandemic highlighted the need for nurses to have more than a working knowledge of ethical principles, an understanding of the characteristics of an ethical dilemma, and the ability to accurately apply the ethical decision-making process. Regarding a differentiation of values, morals, and ethics, Black (2023) indicated that **values** might be viewed as the beliefs of an individual or a group that would be used in guiding behavior, whereas **morals** are rules of conduct that would be used in making a decision regarding right and wrong. The American Nurses Association Professional Nursing Model views nursing as being based on values such as caring, compassion, trustworthiness, acceptance, and accountability, which are derived from beliefs about nursing practice.

The National League for Nursing has established four core values that it views as being most intrinsic to nursing education:

- Caring—promoting health, healing, and hope based on the person's condition.
- Integrity—respect for the dignity and morality of the person without considering potential limitations.
- Diversity—affirms the uniqueness of the person's ideas, values, and ethnic origin.
- Excellence—using ingenuity to create and implement strategies that can be transformational for the individual.[1]

In comparison, **ethics** will reflect the actions that a person should take. An offshoot of this is **bioethics**, meaning the application of ethical principles to the problems that nurses face in healthcare. It is critical that all nurses recognize that, as members of a profession, they must allow their personal morals and values to be overshadowed by the professional ethics articulated by the American Nurses' Association. The ANA has indicated that the *Code of Ethics for Nurses* is nonnegotiable and that each nurse is obligated to uphold it (Black, 2023).

There are two major types of ethical theories that can be used to guide the values and moral behavior of nurses. These are referred to as deontology and consequentialism.

Deontology is based on the rules that allow us to recognize right and wrong actions. Deontology is affiliated with the philosopher Immanuel Kant, who believed that there are universal moral laws that prohibit specific actions such as lying and stealing and that ethical actions will follow these moral laws. This ethical theory involves very little uncertainty since it would require a nurse only to follow the rules as he or she is

---

1. Kimberly Ernstmeyer and Elizabeth Christman, Selections from "Ethical Practice," *Nursing Management and Professional Concepts*, pp. 219, 233–235, Chippewa Valley Technical College. Copyright © 2022 by Kimberly Ernstmeyer and Elizabeth Christman (CC BY 4.0) at https://www.ncbi.nlm.nih.gov/books/NBK598377/.

aware of them and consequently follow through with their professional duty (Ernstmeyer & Christman, 2022).

In comparison, **consequentialism** is an ethical theory that nurses can use to determine whether an action should be implemented based on the potential consequences of the action. For example, consequentialism indicates that although stealing is wrong, if a human life can be saved through the theft of medication, the action is acceptable. A variation on this is **utilitarianism**, which judges the worth of an action by looking at the number of people served positively by that action. Utilitarianism considers healthcare resources such as clinician time and energy, as well as money, as being available in limited amounts that will require allocation based on what society requires (Ernstmeyer & Christman, 2022). Table 1.1 shows a comparison of various ethical issues based on how they are viewed by deontological and consequential theories.

TABLE 1.1 COMPARISON OF ETHICAL ISSUES AS VIEWED BY DEONTOLOGICAL AND CONSEQUENTIAL THEORIES

Ethical Issue	Deontological View	Consequential View
abortion	Unacceptable because life must be preserved.	Abortion may be acceptable in cases of an unwanted pregnancy, rape, incest, or risk to the mother.
stealing	Unacceptable because you are taking something that belongs to another person.	Could be acceptable if stolen goods are redistributed to poor individuals.
killing	Unacceptable because it is always wrong to take a human life.	May be acceptable to take a life in self-defense or if the person who is killed intended to cause harm to others.
physician-assisted suicide	Unacceptable because it is always wrong to end another person's life prematurely.	If a competent adult intends to end his or her life, it should be allowed.
vaccines	Vaccination is a personal choice that may be influenced by factors such as religious beliefs.	Recommended vaccines should be mandatory unless medically contraindicated because of the benefit to the public.

The idea that nurses should be prepared to practice in an ethical manner was initially clarified by Lystra Gretter, the principal of the Farrand

Training School for Nurses and the author of what is now commonly thought of as the **Nightingale pledge**. Although the pledge has fallen out of favor due to its emphasis on loyalty to the physician, it expressed a commitment to the safety and security of the patient and the necessity of holding confidential patient personal information. The pledge in its entirety is stated thus:

> I solemnly pledge myself before God and in the presence of this assembly:
>
> To pass my life in purity and to practice my profession faithfully. I will abstain from whatever is deleterious and mischievous, and will not take or knowingly administer any harmful drug. I will do all in my power to elevate the standard of my profession, and will hold in confidence all personal matters committed to my keeping, and all family affairs coming to my knowledge in the practice of my profession. With loyalty will I endeavor to aid the physician in his work and devote myself to the welfare of those committed to my care. (as cited in Fowler, 2015)

Although the need for a formal code of ethics for nurses was acknowledged as a goal of the newly organized American Nurses Association in 1896, more pressing challenges such as the need to register nurses and the necessity of accrediting schools of nursing initially took precedence. It was not until 1926 that the ANA produced a suggested ethical code that outlined ethical behaviors for nurses. The "suggested" code had progressed into a "tentative" code by 1940, and by 1950 the first formal *Code for Professional Nurses* was adopted by the ANA (Epstein & Turner, 2015).

Holding all nurses to be accountable to the same ethical code serves to protect patients by establishing a standard that nurses will use in implementing ethical decision-making. Each nurse is obligated to clarify his or her own morals and values. When the nurse is clear on his or her personal values, the nurse can recognize and potentially circumvent work situations that might result in a conflict between personal values and professional ethics. When the nurse critically analyzes his or her personal beliefs, morals, and actions, **moral reflection** takes place and the nurse develops moral integrity (Black, 2023). As moral reflection occurs and moral integrity begins to develop, **ethical competence** also begins to grow and develop. This means that the nurse can recognize a potentially ethically challenging situation and can consider different courses of action (Wocial, as cited in Ulrich & Tau, 2012).

The *Code of Ethics for Nurses* is considered to be a "living" document that is regularly updated to reflect societal change. In according with this expectation, by 1968 the code had added interpretations that might assist the nurse to see how the provisions might be applied. The most recent revision of the code as of this writing took place in 2015. The current ***Code of Ethics for Nurses With Interpretive Statements*** is essential for nurses to use in making decisions about their professional conduct in modern society. As previously mentioned, the ethical standard that has been established by the current code is considered to be nonnegotiable by the American Nurses Association and stretches across all roles and healthcare settings. Written by nurses who recognize the professional's commitment to society, the code describes the nursing profession's values and obligations, as well as the duties and professional ideals of the individual nurse. As healthcare continues to become more challenging and nurses gain greater capability to practice across multiple settings simultaneously using multistate licenses, the *Code of Ethics for Nurses* becomes more valuable as a guide to avoid potential ethical land mines in the nursing practice arena (Epstein & Turner, 2015).

The *Code of Ethics for Nurses* of the American Nurses Association consists of nine provisions, which are briefly summarized below. It is recommended that each nurse review the document in its entirety to achieve the greatest understanding of the ethical code's concepts.

TABLE 1.2 SUMMARY OF THE ANA NURSING CODE OF ETHICS BY TOPIC

Provision	Topic	Summary
1	Basic values of the nurse	The nurse practices with compassion and respect for the inherent dignity, worth, and individuality of each person.
2	Commitment of the nurse	The nurse's primary commitment is to the client, whether this is an individual, family, group, community, or population.
3	Protecting the rights of the client	The nurse promotes, advocates for, and protects the rights, health, and safety of the client.
4	Authority, accountability, and responsibility of the nurse	The nurse has authority, accountability, and responsibility for nursing practice; makes decisions; and takes action that is consistent with the obligation to promote health and provide optimal care.

(Continued)

TABLE 1.2 (*Continued*)

Provision	Topic	Summary
5	Duty to self and duty to the individual patient	The nurse owes the same duties to self as to others, including the responsibility to promote health and safety, preserve wholeness of character and integrity, maintain competence, and continue personal and professional growth.
6	Improving the ethical environment	The nurse, through individual and collective effort, establishes, maintains, and improves the ethical environment of the work setting as well as the conditions of employment that will produce safe, quality healthcare.
7	Advancement of the profession	The nurse, in all roles and settings, advances the profession through research and scholarly inquiry, development of professional standards, and the creation of both nursing and health policy.
8	Collaboration with others	The nurse collaborates with health professionals as well as the public to protect human rights, promote health diplomacy, and reduce health disparities.
9	Responsibility of the profession of nursing	The profession of nursing, collectively through its professional organizations, must articulate nursing values, maintain the profession's integrity, and integrate principles of social justice into nursing and health policy.

American Nurses Association, Selection from "Contents," *Code of Ethics for Nurses*, pp. vii–ix. Copyright © 2022 by American Nurses Association; and Marsha Fowler, *Guide to the Code of Ethics for Nurses with Interpretive Statements: Development, Interpretation, and Application*. Copyright © 2015 by American Nurses Association.

NINE PROVISIONS OF THE ANA *CODE OF ETHICS FOR NURSES*

- **Provision 1:** The nurse practices with compassion and respect for the inherent dignity, worth, and unique attributes of every person.
- **Provision 2:** The nurse's primary commitment is to the client, whether an individual, family, group, community, or population.
- **Provision 3:** The nurse promotes, advocates for, and protects the rights, health, and safety of the client.
- **Provision 4:** The nurse has authority, accountability, and responsibility for nursing practice; makes decisions; and takes action

consistent with the obligation to promote health and to provide optimal care.

- **Provision 5:** The nurse owes the same duties to self as to others, including the responsibility to promote health and safety, preserve wholeness of character and integrity, maintain competence, and continue personal and professional growth.
- **Provision 6:** The nurse, through individual and collective effort, establishes, maintains, and improves the ethical environment of the work setting and conditions of employment that are conducive to safe, quality healthcare.
- **Provision 7:** The nurse, in all roles and settings, advances the profession through research and scholarly inquiry, professional standards development, and the generation of both nursing and health policy.
- **Provision 8:** The nurse collaborates with other health professionals and the public to protect human rights, promote health diplomacy, and reduce health disparities.
- **Provision 9:** The profession of nursing, collectively through its professional organizations, must articulate nursing values, maintain the integrity of the profession, and integrate principles of social justice into nursing and health policy.[2]

In summary, the *Code of Ethics for Nurses* of the American Nurses' Association serves to guide the modern nurse through the ethical maze that engulfs healthcare in general and the nursing profession specifically. Although the ANA *Code of Ethics for Nurses* can serve as a map for today's practitioner, it becomes easier to utilize when each nurse has a sufficient background in ethical principles. These will be discussed in the subsequent chapter.

REFERENCES

Black, B. P. (2023). *Professional nursing: Concepts & challenges*. Elsevier Health Sciences.

Epstein, B., & Turner, M. (May 31, 2015). "The Nursing Code of Ethics: Its value, its history." *OJIN: The Online Journal of Issues in Nursing, 20*(2), Manuscript 4.

Ernstmeyer K., & Christman E. (Eds.). (2022). *Nursing management and professional Concepts*. Open Resources for Nursing (Open RN). https://www.ncbi.nlm.nih.gov/books/NBK598377/.

2. Marsha Fowler, *Guide to the Code of Ethics for Nurses with Interpretive Statements: Development, Interpretation, and Application*. Copyright © 2015 by American Nurses Association.

Fowler, M. D. M. (2015). *Guide to the Code of Ethics for Nurses with Interpretive Statements: Development, interpretation, and application*. American Nurses Association.
Ulrich, C. M., & Tau, T. (2012). *Nursing ethics in everyday practice*. Sigma Theta Tau International.

NCLEX FORMAT REVIEW QUESTIONS

1. Choose the statements that are most applicable to a deontological ethical view. (Select all that apply)

   a. _____ Based on the rules that allow the nurse to recognize right and wrong actions

   b. _____ Can be used to determine whether an action should be implemented based on the potential consequences of the action

   c. _____ Involves little uncertainty since it would require a nurse only to follow the rules and consequently follow through with professional duty

   d. _____ Judges the worth of an action by looking at the number of people served positively by that action

   e. _____ Considers healthcare resources that will require allocation based on what society requires

   f. _____ Based on the idea that there are universal moral laws that prohibit specific actions

   g. _____ Based on the idea that ethical actions will follow moral laws

answer: a, c, f, g

2. Choose the statements that are most applicable to a consequential ethical view. (Select all that apply)

   a. _____ Based on the rules that allow the nurse to recognize right and wrong actions

   b. _____ Can be used to determine whether an action should be implemented based on the potential consequences of the action

   c. _____ Involves little uncertainty since it would require a nurse only to follow the rules and consequently follow through with professional duty

d. _____ Judges the worth of an action by looking at the number of people served positively by that action

e. _____ Considers healthcare resources that will require allocation based on what society requires

f. _____ Based on the idea that there are universal moral laws that prohibit specific actions

g. _____ Based on the idea that ethical actions will follow moral laws

answer: b, d, e

3. The provision of the *Code of Ethics for Nurses* of the American Nurses Association that concerns collaboration with other health professionals is:

   a. _____ provision 6

   b. _____ provision 7

   c. _____ provision 8

   d. _____ provision 9

answer: c

4. The provision of the *Code of Ethics for Nurses* of the American Nurses Association that concerns the need to protect the rights of the client is:

   a. _____ provision 1

   b. _____ provision 2

   c. _____ provision 3

   d. _____ provision 4

answer: c

5. The core value of the National League for Nursing that involves the uniqueness of the client's ideas, values, and ethnic origin is:

   a. _____ diversity

   b. _____ caring

   c. _____ integrity

   d. _____ excellence

answer: a

TEAM-BUILDING EXERCISE

Instructions: Divide students into teams of at least three people and preferably no more than five. Each person should have a role assigned in the exercise. One person will be the leader, one person will be the timekeeper, and one person will be the recorder. The **leader** will oversee helping the discussion progress so that the objectives of the exercise are accomplished. The **timekeeper** should intervene when necessary to keep the discussion focused on the topic of the exercise and should periodically remind team members of the amount of time remaining to complete the exercise. The **recorder** will be responsible for taking notes during the discussion that can be utilized when the exercise results are presented to the class. If additional team members are included in the group, one person can be assigned to assist with the note-taking and transcription process, and the additional person can assist the team leader in guiding the discussion and assist in preparing the final presentation of the results.

SCENARIO FOR TEAM-BUILDING EXERCISE

Ruth is a registered nurse who works the 7:00 p.m. to 7:00 a.m. shift on the surgical stepdown floor. As you arrive for work one morning, you see her sitting in the nurse manager's office crying. One of the other nurses excitedly tells you that Ruth is being fired from her position for stealing narcotics out of the floor's medication room. The nurse tells you that Ruth was heard telling the nurse manager that she was using the narcotics to help her sister who is dying from a particularly painful form of cancer and is unemployed.

QUESTIONS

1. How would deontology view this as an ethical situation? Be able to explain your position.

2. How would consequentialism view this as an ethical situation? Be able to explain your position.

3. Which provision(s) of the ANA *Code of Ethics for Nurses* do you view as being most applicable to this situation? Be able to explain your position.

4. Which values included in the American Nurses Association's Professional Nursing Model do you view as being exemplified by this situation? Be able to explain your position.

CHAPTER 2

ETHICAL PRINCIPLES

CHAPTER OBJECTIVES

After studying this chapter, students will be able to:

- Define autonomy as an ethical principle and discuss its relationship to patient care.
- Define beneficence as an ethical principle and discuss its relationship to patient care.
- Define fidelity as an ethical principle and discuss its relationship to patient care.
- Define justice as an ethical principle and discuss its relationship to patient care.
- Define nonmaleficence as an ethical principle and discuss its relationship to patient care.
- Define veracity as an ethical principle and discuss its relationship to patient care.
- Describe the various aspects of the Patient Self-Determination Act.
- Discuss the various aspects of soft and hard paternalism.
- Describe the principle of double effect.
- Discuss the differences between distributive justice and social justice.
- Describe how equality differs from fairness.
- Discuss the consequences of failing to practice fidelity.
- Describe the difference between beneficence and nonmaleficence.
- Discuss negligence and its relationship to nonmaleficence.
- Describe how an informed consent for treatment relates to the principle of autonomy.

KEY TERMS

advance directive
autonomy
beneficence
distributive justice

double effect
equality
fairness
fidelity
justice
hard paternalism
informed consent
nonmaleficence
paternalism
Patient Self-Determination Act
social justice
soft paternalism
veracity

As modern life has become more complex, the ethical decision-making process nurses must engage in has consequently become more difficult. In order for nurses to be as prepared as possible for this, a thorough understanding of the ethical principles that form the basis for ethical decision-making must be incorporated. Black (2023) has indicated that human dignity and a respect for persons are foundational to the basic ethical principles of autonomy, beneficence, nonmaleficence, justice, fidelity, and veracity.

AUTONOMY

Butts and Rich (2020) describe **autonomy** as the freedom and ability to act in a manner that is self-determined; this means that the individual can make a personal decision without outside interference and anticipates that the decision will be honored.

In the healthcare arena, the principle of autonomy is being utilized when

- an **informed consent** for treatment is obtained, meaning that the patient has received the information that a reasonable person would need to know about the procedure, was not coerced to provide consent, and was competent to understand the information;
- a patient's wishes regarding treatment options are honored, even if the medical team does not necessarily agree with the patient's choices;
- privacy and confidentiality are maintained; and
- the medical team is truthful in providing a patient with comprehensive information on a diagnosis and treatment options.

An individual's autonomy is typically curtailed if the person becomes a threat to others, such as implementing acts of violence. An individual's autonomous decision, such as a consent for treatment, for example, will be based on the following:

- the values of the person

- having sufficient information to make an informed decision
- a lack of coercion to make a decision
- the ability to use reason and to deliberate in making a decision (Black, 2023)

A respect for the autonomy of the patient can be lacking in healthcare when providers automatically assume that an older adult's children should be involved in making decisions about the parent's healthcare, or when an assumption is made that a patient's mental status is deteriorating simply because his or her physical condition has changed.

A piece of legislation that is directly linked to the right to autonomy is the **Patient Self-Determination Act**, which was passed by Congress in 1990. It gives patients the legal right to determine whether they want every type of heroic measure to be taken in the event of a life-or-death situation and requires hospitals to honor the patient's wishes regarding the **advance directive**, which is the legal document indicating the wishes of the person pertaining to end-of-life care (Black, 2023).

BENEFICENCE

While adhering to the principle of autonomy means that the rights of the individual are respected regarding his or her choices, the principle of **beneficence** recognizes the need for the nurse to always act in a way that is in the best interest of the patient. This is particularly important when the patient may not be able to verbalize his or her need for assistance, such as a request for pain medication (Ulrich, 2012). Beauchamp and Childress (2019) have indicated that there are at least five rules that are included as part of the practice of beneficence:

- protecting and defending the rights of the individual
- preventing harm from occurring to the person
- removing any condition that is believed to cause harm to another person
- assisting individuals with disabilities
- rescuing individuals believed to be in danger

The actions involved in the practice of beneficence should always be considered in light of the patient's overall situation to ensure that they do not conflict with his or her values and beliefs. For example, both the patient and the nurse may agree that the patient needs to get more sleep at night. Although the nurse initially may consider speaking with the physician regarding use of a sleep medication, the patient might choose to avoid this treatment option, preferring to utilize natural sleeping aids. Therefore, the nurse would research the various homeopathic remedies that might be recommended for the patient in an effort to assist the patient (Black, 2023).

Once the nurse recognizes that the principle of beneficence can conflict with the principle of autonomy, the challenge becomes to avoid **paternalism**. This occurs when the patient is not allowed to exercise autonomy because the nurse perceives a greater need to exercise beneficence. An example of paternalism would be if the nurse decided not to inform a patient about changes in his or her vital signs for fear that the patient would show symptoms of further anxiety. Beauchamp and Childress (2019) have identified two types of paternalism:

- **soft paternalism**: this type of paternalism attempts to protect the person from his or her own involuntary conduct. This typically occurs when the patient is unable to make reasonable decisions due to substance abuse or mental illness.
- **hard paternalism**: this type of paternalism attempts to protect a patient who is making risky choices, despite his or her actions being informed and voluntary. This typically occurs when the patient is at risk for significant harm that could be preventable.

The nurse may need to assume the role of advocate for the patient if family members attempt to practice paternalism. An example of this would be if family members tried to convince the patient's medical team to avoid telling the patient that he or she has a terminal condition for fear that the patient would become suicidal.

NONMALEFICENCE

Closely related to the principle of beneficence is that of **nonmaleficence**, which literally means to avoid actions that cause harm. This does not apply to situations such as the administration of chemotherapy, which may include a risk of harm for the patient but may eventually produce the greater good of arresting the spread of a cancerous tumor. Black (2023) identifies the principle that justifies the risk of harm to the patient as **double effect**. The principle of double effect indicates that it is ethically permissible for the nurse to produce a distressing effect on the patient if the intent is to ultimately produce an overall positive effect for the person. Beauchamp and Childress (2019) have identified several issues that are associated with the principle of nonmaleficence:

- upholding standards of due care—this means that the nurse abides by the standards that are specific to nursing and provides the expected care that a reasonable person in the nursing profession would provide.
- avoiding negligence—negligence occurs when the due care that is expected does not take place and there is a risk of harm. The risk of harm can be unintended and careless or intentional and reckless.
- rules pertaining to nontreatment and end-of-life decisions—these include:
    - when to withhold and withdraw life-sustaining treatment
    - when to apply extraordinary treatment
    - when to utilize various types of technology to sustain life
    - the intended effects of a treatment or medication and the merely foreseen effects
    - when to allow a patient to die

JUSTICE

The various emotions of the patient and family members who are facing the need to make difficult treatment decisions, as well as those of their supporting healthcare team, can raise the issue of **justice**. This refers to equality as well as fairness.

Equality means that patients receive comparable treatment without consideration of any type of personal characteristic, whereas **fairness** refers to the distribution of costs, benefits, and risks equally between individuals (Ulrich, 2012). It is expected that patients with the same healthcare needs will receive comparable care. Black (2023) notes that research has indicated that the distribution of resources in the healthcare system is not equitable across racial groups. Butts and Rich (2020) indicated that whereas **distributive justice** refers to the allocation of resources in a fair and equitable manner, **social justice** proposes that benefits and responsibilities should be distributed fairly among all the members of a society. Ideally, all society members would have the same rights, opportunities, and responsibilities regarding healthcare. To ensure some measure of social justice exists regarding healthcare, the Patient Protection and Affordable Care Act was enacted in 2010. The intent of the legislation was to improve the quality of healthcare and lower costs while consequently providing greater access to healthcare. Issues surrounding the Patient Protection and Affordable Care Act included the following:

- Will the legislation be more efficient in providing healthcare or become a casualty of the federal bureaucracy?
- Will the legislation make medicine more rational?
- Is healthcare a right or a privilege?

FIDELITY

The principle of justice includes the idea of distribution of healthcare according to the needs of the consumer. This is a close relative to the principle of **fidelity**. Fidelity pertains to the importance of honoring commitments, specifically in this case those commitments made to patients. The legal system attempts to ensure that nurses will practice with fidelity by requiring that nurses be licensed to practice their profession. The nurse who is licensed as a prerequisite to joining the nursing profession enters into a contract with society and consequently agrees to accept certain responsibilities (Black, 2023).

Ulrich (2012) indicated that the word *fidelity* is synonymous with faithfulness or loyalty. In the nursing profession, fidelity is inclusive of the trust patients place in nurses as a significant part of the healthcare team as well as the reliability and integrity of the treatments being administered. The loyalty or obligation of the nurse is also a significant aspect of fidelity. The nurse has an obligation to the patient and potentially to the patient's family members, to the employing facility, and to colleagues, as well as to the self. It is this principle that causes the nurse to admit when he or she has made an error in patient care.

Faubion (n.d.) indicated that practicing fidelity in nursing can build trust between the patient and the members of the healthcare team, promote the development of positive patient care outcomes, lead to increased patient satisfaction, and facilitate a greater degree of patient autonomy. The practice of fidelity promotes a greater degree of clarity in nurse–patient communication. This improves a patient's ability to follow discharge instructions and can contribute to satisfactory patient care outcomes.

What can be the consequences of failing to practice fidelity? They can include the following:

- Loss of credibility with colleagues
- Disruption to a previously plotted career path, particularly if the failure to practice fidelity results in a job loss or revocation of the nursing license

- Failure of patients to adhere to treatment plans upon discharge, resulting in poor patient care outcomes and decreased patient satisfaction

VERACITY

A close ethical relative of fidelity is **veracity**. Essentially this consists of telling the truth. An integral part of the nurse–patient relationship is the expectation that the nurse will be truthful with his or her patients. This can lay the foundation for an ethical dilemma for the nurse, who may be forced to withhold information from a patient because the physician has not yet spoken with the patient about a diagnosis. An ethical dilemma can also result if the healthcare provider chooses not to provide the patient with information because the provider believes that the patient is not capable of understanding the discussion or should not be informed about his or her condition. This would be indicative of an attitude of paternalism. As discussed under the section on beneficence, this means that the provider believes that he or she knows what is best for the patient even though the patient seems to be competent to make an autonomous decision about healthcare treatment. A similar ethical dilemma can result for the nurse if the patient's family asks that the patient not be informed about a life-threatening diagnosis (Black, 2023).

The American Nurses' Association (2024) has noted that nurse veracity is particularly important is several situations, such as the following:

- Informing a patient about treatment potential side effects; being honest but mindful of the need to avoid alarming patients to such an extent that they choose to cancel potential life-saving treatments such as chemotherapy
- Explaining information from a patient's chart in language that is easily understandable
- Acknowledging errors that were made during treatment

The practice of veracity in nursing is particularly important in the development of a cohesive healthcare team. The nurse should feel comfortable enough with peers and supervisory staff to verbalize if a potential error or safety issue seems likely to occur. Intervening while demonstrating compassion for the colleague can help solidify the healthcare team while avoiding serious injury to the patient.

In summary, the nurse who seeks to navigate the potentially treacherous waters of modern healthcare must have a thorough understanding of the ethical principles that have been presented in this section. A summary of the information regarding the ethical principles is presented in Table 2.1. Once this is achieved, the foundation has been laid to enable the nurse to accurately engage in ethical decision-making. The intricacies of this process will be discussed in the subsequent chapter.

TABLE 2.1 ETHICAL PRINCIPLES

Ethical Principle	Definition	Accompanying Concepts
autonomy	freedom and ability to act in a manner that is self-determined; the individual makes a personal decision without outside interference and anticipates that the decision will be honored	informed consent, Patient Self-Determination Act, advance directive
beneficence	requires the nurse to act in a way that is in the best interest of the patient	soft paternalism, hard paternalism
nonmaleficence	avoid actions that cause harm	double effect, standards of due care, negligence
justice	refers to equality as well as fairness	distributive justice, social justice
fidelity	distribution of healthcare according to the needs of the consumer	faithfulness, loyalty
veracity	telling the truth	paternalism, ethical dilemma

REFERENCES

American Nurses Association. (February 9, 2024). *What is veracity in nursing?* ANA Nursing Resources Hub.

Beauchamp, T., & Childress, J. (2019). *Principles of biomedical ethics*. Oxford University Press.

Black, B. P. (2023). *Professional nursing: Concepts & challenges*. Elsevier Health Sciences.

Butts, J., & Rich, K. (2020). *Nursing ethics: Across the curriculum and into practice*. Jones and Bartlett Learning.

Faubion, D. (n.d.). Fidelity in nursing—What is it, why is it important & examples. Retrieved December 20, 2024, from nursingprocess.org

Ulrich, C. (2012). *Nursing ethics in everyday practice*. Sigma Theta Tau International.

NCLEX FORMAT REVIEW QUESTIONS

1. A patient is experiencing a form of mental illness that leads him to occasionally become violent. The ethical principle that is most likely to be curtailed in this case is:
    a. autonomy
    b. beneficence
    c. nonmaleficence
    d. justice
    e. fidelity
    f. veracity

answer: a

2. The Patient Protection and Affordable Care Act is primarily related to which ethical principle?
    a. autonomy
    b. beneficence
    c. nonmaleficence
    d. justice
    e. fidelity
    f. veracity

answer: d

3. A nurse makes an error when preparing and administering medication. Although the patient was not harmed, the nurse reports the error to the nurse manager and the patient's physician. The nurse is adhering most closely to which ethical principle in this case?
    a. autonomy
    b. beneficence
    c. nonmaleficence
    d. justice
    e. fidelity
    f. veracity

answer: e

4. A patient who has been diagnosed with cancer decides against being treated with chemotherapy. In honoring this wish, the medical team is adhering to the ethical principle of:

   a. autonomy

   b. beneficence

   c. nonmaleficence

   d. justice

   e. fidelity

   f. veracity

answer: a

5. A nurse makes certain to return to check on their patient at 9:00 p.m. as promised. In honoring this promise to the patient, the nurse is adhering to which ethical principle?

   a. autonomy

   b. beneficence

   c. nonmaleficence

   d. justice

   e. fidelity

   f. veracity

answer: e

6. A patient asks their nurse about the latest blood pressure reading that was assessed when vital signs were taken. The nurse provides this information because he is adhering to the ethical principle of:

   a. autonomy

   b. beneficence

   c. nonmaleficence

   d. justice

   e. fidelity

   f. veracity

answer: f

7. A patient has been diagnosed with terminal cancer. Her family asks the medical team not to tell the patient about her diagnosis

for fear that she will become depressed and lose hope. This is an example of:

a. distributive justice
b. paternalism
c. double effect
d. fairness
e. nonmaleficence
f. equality

answer: b

8. A home health nurse ensures that all of his patients receive comparable treatment without considering any of the patients' personal characteristics. The nurse is adhering to which principle?

a. distributive justice
b. paternalism
c. double effect
d. fairness
e. nonmaleficence
f. equality

answer: f

9. A physician explains to their patient that the chemotherapy that has been ordered will produce significant side effects that could even be life-threatening. However, these are the only drugs known to be effective against the patient's particular form of cancer. This is an example of:

a. distributive justice
b. paternalism
c. double effect
d. fairness
e. nonmaleficence
f. equality

answer: c

10. A nurse ensures that he maintains the standards that are specific to nursing and provides the expected care that any reasonable nurse would provide. This is associated with which ethical principle?
    a. distributive justice
    b. paternalism
    c. double effect
    d. fairness
    e. nonmaleficence
    f. equality

answer: e

TEAM-BUILDING EXERCISE

Instructions: Divide students into teams of at least three people and preferably no more than five. Each person should have a role assigned in the exercise. One person will be the leader, one person will be the timekeeper, and one person will be the recorder. The **leader** will oversee helping the discussion progress so that the objectives of the exercise are accomplished. The **timekeeper** should intervene when necessary to keep the discussion focused on the topic of the exercise and should periodically remind team members of the amount of time remaining to complete the exercise. The **recorder** will be responsible for taking notes during the discussion that can be utilized when the exercise results are presented to the class. If additional team members are included in the group, one person can be assigned to assist with the note-taking and transcription process, and the additional person can assist the team leader in guiding the discussion and assist in preparing the final presentation of the results.

SCENARIO FOR TEAM-BUILDING EXERCISE

You are caring for Mrs. Jones, a patient who has been undergoing testing to determine the cause of her persistent abdominal pain. As you are conducting your assessments of your patients, Mrs. Jones's family stops you before you can enter her room. Mrs. Jones's daughter tells you tearfully that the physician has told the family that Mrs. Jones's pain is caused by a return of her colon cancer, which will most likely be terminal. The daughter tells you that the physician has not told Mrs.

Jones about the diagnosis at the family's request and that the family does not want her to know for fear that she will become depressed and lose hope of a recovery.

QUESTIONS

1. How does this situation violate the ethical principle of autonomy?

2. How does this situation violate the ethical principle of beneficence?

3. How does this situation serve as an example of paternalism?

4. Which aspects of the situation relate to the ethical principle of nonmaleficence? Do you view the principle as being upheld or violated? Explain your answer.

5. Which aspects of the situation violate the ethical principle of veracity?

CHAPTER 3

ETHICAL DECISION-MAKING

CHAPTER OBJECTIVES

After studying this chapter, students will be able to:

- Identify and explain the steps in the process of ethical decision-making.
- Discuss how to clarify an existing ethical dilemma.
- Discuss how to identify the various alternatives that could be implemented in an ethical dilemma.
- Identify the three tests to determine whether the best option has been selected for resolution of an ethical dilemma.
- Describe common types of ethical dilemmas that can occur in healthcare.
- Discuss ethical dilemmas that occurred as a result of the COVID-19 pandemic.
- Discuss Jonsen's Four Topics Method for ethical analysis.
- Discuss the purpose and the various goals of an ethics committee.

KEY TERMS

advance directive
ethical decision-making
ethical dilemma
ethics committee
healthcare power of attorney
Jonsen's Four Topics Method for ethical analysis
values

Every day, nurses encounter situations that require them to implement interventions that are based on their professional judgments. The ethical decisions are made through collaboration with the patient, his or her support system, and various members of the healthcare team.

All the perspectives held by these individuals must be considered as the nurse makes a decision. The process of **ethical decision-making** means that the nurse sometimes makes a professional judgment when two or more values seem to be incongruent. **Values** are learned beliefs that help an individual choose an option when there are multiple alternatives, none of which seem to be an appropriate selection. Initially, a person's values are formed by the beliefs, attitudes, qualities, and religious views of their childhood caregivers, and these values continue to develop as the person is exposed to influences from friends and family members. As previously discussed, the values for a profession form the profession's code of ethics. When the nurse's personal or professional values seem to conflict with the options that are available, an **ethical dilemma** results. It is important to recognize that the "best" decision must be made in this case, since in a true ethical dilemma, there typically will not be an obvious right or wrong answer (Black, 2023).

COMMON TYPES OF ETHICAL DILEMMAS

Several types of ethical dilemmas can result when the nurse's personal values conflict with professional values. These include but are not limited to the following.

Dilemmas involving the behavior of other professionals. Conflict can develop due to a member of the healthcare team failing to meet the established standard of care through incompetent behavior or through actions that are considered to be unethical by the other team members, such as failing to respect the patient's right to autonomy. Such an ethical dilemma can easily result from careless use of social media. A nurse or other healthcare team member must not post anything pertaining to a patient that could violate the right to privacy and confidentiality. Be aware that the patient's right to privacy is not necessarily ensured by the privacy settings applicable to various forms of social media. Posting photographs of patients must be avoided as must online contact with patients. It cannot be overemphasized that a digital "footprint" is created through the posting of any type of entry that cannot be eliminated. Another type of ethical dilemma that falls under this category is the decision of when to confront a colleague who is clearly dependent on drugs or alcohol. This can include prescription medications if they are negatively affecting the person's ability to provide patient care that meets ethical standards. It is important for the nurse who recognizes that such behavior is occurring to confront the colleague promptly to prevent an injury from occurring to the patient and to assist the impaired colleague from sustaining discipline to their license. Guidelines on how to implement this process and the options that are available to the impaired nurse are available through each state's board of nursing website.

Dilemmas involving patients' rights. As previously discussed in an earlier chapter, the patient is now recognized as the most important member of the healthcare team, with the right to autonomy in decision-making as well as the right to confidentiality. Healthcare team members must determine whether patients have completed an **advance directive**; this is a legal document that indicates the person's wishes regarding end-of-life issues when the person is critically ill. Also, the team member must determine whether **healthcare power of attorney** has been assigned. This means that an individual trusted by the patient has been appointed to make decisions related to healthcare for the person when the patient cannot make them unassisted. Conflict can easily occur when family members are not aware of the appointment of an individual holding healthcare power of attorney and all members wish to provide input on the patient's situation.

ETHICAL DILEMMAS THAT DEVELOPED DURING THE PANDEMIC

Ethical dilemmas that many nurses had never faced before developed as the recent pandemic appeared on the national scene and quickly reached a crisis level. These included the following.

Allocation of scarce resources—decisions were suddenly needing to be made by health are teams regarding which patients should be allocated a ventilator out of their facility's dwindling supply, how healthcare could be prioritized among the increasing throng of patients, and how patients could most accurately have their prognosis determined.

Personal protection equipment—as clinicians began to face the possibility of having to practice without having adequate personal protection equipment and potentially risking their own lives to care for patients, the dilemma arose regarding when a provider could legitimately judge that the risk to the clinician's own safety was greater than the benefit that could be provided to the patient.

Availability of a vaccine—clinicians were faced with the need to ensure an adequate supply of a vaccine that had not undergone the usual rigorous testing that had previously been considered standard for such a substance. Also, a secondary ethical dilemma emerged when nurses, cautious about utilizing such an undertested substance themselves, refused to take the vaccination and were terminated from their positions, thus further straining a workforce already at a crisis level (Chamsi-Pasha et al., 2020).

PROCESS OF ETHICAL DECISION-MAKING

There are several steps that are used in the process of ethical decision-making.

Clarify the existing ethical dilemma. Determine what is the specific issue at the root of the dilemma. Who will make the final decision? Determine all the stakeholders who will be affected by the dilemma as well as the final decision. Specify the value conflicts that exist as well as the time frame that is given for coming to a decision. Ulrich (2012) notes that a dilemma frequently concerns moral values and therefore will be individualized. Although most societies adhere to a set of common moral values, the importance that is given to a specific value is unique to each person. This means that when a dilemma involves a moral issue, there must be a choice made between various alternatives to implement as well as a selection of the value associated with that alternative.

Gather additional data needed. Reiner (2022) recommends verifying that the issue is truly an ethical one and not a legal one. Determine whether there are any legal precedents that relate to the situation, since ethical and legal issues can coexist. If there are legal aspects involved (such as would be present when a patient is potentially being removed from life support), make certain that the facility's risk management department has been consulted. In addition, apply the *Code of Ethics for Nurses* to the issue to gain additional information for use in coming to a decision (this will be discussed in detail in the subsequent chapter).

Identify existing options. Determine all the available alternative solutions that exist. Work with the previously identified stakeholders as well as the patient, support system, and the members of the healthcare team to identify as many options as possible to ensure that an acceptable solution will be found. Which solutions are viewed as being most feasible? Which solutions would be most difficult to implement? Clarify the factors that would make the solutions difficult to carry out to verify that there are legitimate barriers present.

Make a decision. Review each identified option and determine the potential impact of each one. Review ethical principles (see Chapter 2) to determine the significance of each option being considered. Recognize that attempting to avoid the responsibility attached to making such a decision is not an option.

Implement the actions associated with the decision. Implement the course of action that has been selected. Continue to collaborate with the various members of the healthcare team, the patient, and the support system to ensure that implementation progresses smoothly.

Evaluate the decisions and the implemented actions. Since a crisis situation frequently precipitates an ethical dilemma, unexpected outcomes can occur. Reflect on the decision that was made to determine whether a different course of action might have resulted in better outcomes. At this point, if the ethical dilemma has not been resolved, make certain that the issue at hand has been clarified—the true dilemma will be the patient's right to autonomy versus the nurse's professional ethics and conflicting personal beliefs. Determine whether additional data are available that were not previously identified and then reevaluate to identify the existing alternatives (Black, 2023). Reiner (2022) recommends applying three "tests" for determining whether the best option has been selected:

- test of justice: the nurse should consider his or her own sense of fairness; would the nurse treat others the same in a similar situation?
- test of publicity: would the nurse want his or her behavior in this situation reported in the media?
- test of universality: would the nurse recommend the same course of action to another nurse?

TABLE 3.1 PROCESS OF ETHICAL DECISION-MAKING

Step	Description
Clarify the existing ethical dilemma	Determine the specific issue at the root of the dilemma. Determine all stakeholders who will be affected by the dilemma and the final decision. Specify value conflicts and the time frame that exists for coming to a decision.
Gather additional data needed.	Determine legal precedents that relate to the situation. If there are legal aspects involved, ensure that the risk management department has been consulted. Apply the *Code of Ethics for Nurses*.

(*Continued*)

TABLE 3.1 *(Continued)*

Step	Description
Identify existing options.	Determine available alternative solutions. Work with stakeholders to identify as many options as possible to ensure that an acceptable solution will be found. Which solutions are most feasible? Which solutions would be most difficult to implement? Clarify the factors that would make the solutions difficult to implement.
Make a decision.	Review each identified option and determine the potential impact of each. Review ethical principles to determine the significance of each option. Attempting to avoid the responsibility attached to making a decision is not an option.
Implement actions associated with the decision.	Implement selected course of action. Collaborate with the healthcare team, patient, and support system to ensure that implementation progresses smoothly. Evaluate decisions and the implemented actions. Since a crisis can precipitate an ethical dilemma, unexpected outcomes can occur. Reflect on the decision to determine whether a different course of action might have resulted in better outcomes. Apply tests to determine whether the best option has been selected: ▸ test of justice: would the nurse treat others the same in a similar situation? ▸ test of publicity: would the nurse want his or her behavior in this situation reported in the media? ▸ test of universality: would the nurse recommend the same course of action to another nurse?

JONSEN'S FOUR TOPICS METHOD

Another approach to ethical decision-making involves **Jonsen's Four Topics Method for ethical analysis** (Jonsen et al., 2015). The healthcare team will gather all the relevant information regarding a specific patient case and will progress toward a resolution by using a structured analytic process. The patient's case will be analyzed using four topics: medical indications, patient preferences, quality of life, and contextual features. This method encourages communication between the patient, members of the support network, and the healthcare team while also incorporating the ethical principles of beneficence, nonmaleficence, autonomy, and justice. To gather the relevant information, the healthcare team will attempt to answer specific questions in each of the four areas:

- Medical indications
  - What is the patient's specific medical problem?
  - What are the identified goals of treatment?
  - Are there circumstances in which medical treatments would not be indicated?
  - Which treatment option is most likely to be successful?
  - How can the patient benefit from medical and nursing care? How can harm to the patient be avoided?
- Patient preferences
  - Has the patient been informed of the benefits and risk of medical treatment, indicated understanding of the information, and provided consent?
  - Is the patient both mentally and legally competent to provide consent?
  - Has the patient stated preferences about treatment?
  - If the patient is now incapacitated and cannot provide consent, did he or she express preferences regarding treatment in the past?
  - If the patient is now incapacitated and cannot provide consent, who is the appropriate surrogate to make decisions regarding treatment?
  - Is the patient unwilling to cooperate with the recommended medical treatment? If so, why?
- Quality of life
  - What are the patient's prospects for a return to normal life with treatment? What are the prospects for such a return without treatment? Is the patient likely to experience physical, mental, and/or social deficits even if treatment is judged to be successful?
  - How could a judgment be made regarding the quality of life that would be desirable or undesirable for a patient who either cannot make such a judgment or cannot express such a judgment?
  - Are there biases that could prejudice the healthcare provider's evaluation of the patient's quality of life either positively or negatively?
  - Are there ethical issues that can occur regarding either improving or enhancing the patient's quality of life?

- Do the assessments on quality of life raise questions regarding a possible change in treatment plan, such as a need to forgo life-sustaining treatment?
- What is the legal and ethical status of suicide, if the patient is considering this?

- Contextual features
  - Are there professional, interprofessional, or business interests that could create conflicts of interest regarding patients' treatment?
  - Are there individuals other than members of the healthcare team or the patient, such as family members, who are interested in clinical decisions?
  - Are there third parties with legitimate interests that could legitimately impose limits on patient confidentiality?
  - Are there identified financial factors that will create conflicts of interest as clinical decisions are made?
  - Are there problems associated with the allocation of scarce health resources that will influence clinical decisions?
  - Are there religious issues that could influence clinical decisions?
  - Are there legal issues that could influence clinical decisions?
  - Are there considerations related to clinical research and education that could influence clinical decisions?
  - Are there issues related to public safety and public health that could influence clinical decisions?
  - Are there potential conflicts of interest within organizations that could influence clinical decisions and affect the welfare of the patient?

The Four Topics approach allows the members of the healthcare team to place the facts of a patient's case in a structured format and facilitate the critical thinking process regarding ethical dilemmas.

TABLE 3.2 JONSEN'S FOUR TOPICS METHOD

Topic	Questions
Medical indications	What is the patient's medical problem? What are the goals of treatment? In which circumstances would medical treatments not be indicated? Which treatment option is most likely to be successful? How will the patient benefit from medical and nursing care? How can harm to the patient be prevented?

Topic	**Questions**
Patient preferences	Has the patient been informed of benefits and risks of medical treatment and provided consent?
	Is the patient both mentally and legally competent to provide consent?
	Does the patient have preferences about treatment?
	If the patient cannot provide consent now, did he or she express preferences regarding treatment in the past?
	If the patient cannot provide consent now, who is the surrogate to make decisions regarding treatment?
	Is the patient unwilling to cooperate with medical treatment? If so, why?
Quality of life	What are the patient's prospects for a return to normal life with treatment?
	Could normal life resume without treatment?
	Is the patient likely to experience physical, mental, or social deficits even with successful treatment?
	How can a judgment be made about quality of life for a patient who cannot either make or express such a judgment?
	Which biases could prejudice the nurse's evaluation of the patient's quality of life?
	Are there ethical issues that can occur regarding improving the patient's quality of life?
	Are there questions about a possible change in treatment plans?
	What is the legal and ethical status of suicide, if the patient is considering this?
Contextual features	Are there professional, interprofessional, or business interests that could create conflicts of interest regarding patients' treatment?
	Are there individuals such as family members who are interested in clinical decisions?
	Are there third parties with legitimate interests that could impose limits on patient confidentiality?
	Are there identified financial factors that will create conflicts of interest as clinical decisions are made?
	Are there problems associated with the allocation of scarce health resources that will influence clinical decisions?
	Are there religious issues that could influence clinical decisions?
	Are there legal issues that could influence clinical decisions?
	Are there considerations related to clinical research and education that could influence clinical decisions?
	Are there issues related to public safety and public health that could influence clinical decisions?
	Are there potential conflicts of interest within organizations that could influence clinical decisions, as well as the welfare of the patient?

ETHICS COMMITTEE

Frequently, multifaceted ethical decisions will be made utilizing a team approach. When a team comprises members who assemble on a regular basis to discuss the ethical issues within a facility, it is considered to be an **ethics committee**. The ethics committee may question the patient's ability to make decisions and the support system members' ability to talk with the physician or family. The ethics committee may opt to meet with the patient, family members, support system members, and surrogate decision-maker. Here are the essential goals of an ethics committee:

- Provide support and guidance to patients, support system, and other members of the healthcare team involved in the decision-making process
- Review cases as requested when there appear to be conflicts in values
- Assist in clarifying situations that extend beyond the scope of ordinary practice, particularly those that are ethical or legal in nature
- Help clarify the issue at hand, discuss available and feasible alternatives, and suggest reasonable compromises
- Promote patients' rights
- Assist the patient and support system members in coming to consensus on an option that most appropriately meets the patient's needs
- Promote policies and procedures that would assist in achieving patient-centered outcomes
- Enhance the overall ethical tone of the organizations and professionals involved

In summary, the nurse who continues to practice in the modern post-COVID healthcare environment can expect to be faced with healthcare dilemmas that are unique to this time in history, as well as those that have confronted nurses since the profession began. The question of how to practice nursing in the most ethical manner possible while skillfully dodging obstacles to ethical decision-making will continue to plague clinicians. The subsequent chapter will address how to utilize the American Nurses Association's *Code of Ethics for Nurses* to guide ethical practice.

REFERENCES

Black, B. P. (2023). *Professional nursing: Concepts & challenges*. Elsevier Health Sciences.

Chamsi-Pasha, H., Chamsi-Pasha, M., & Albar, M. (2020). Ethical dilemmas in the era of COVID-19. *Avicenna Journal of Medicine*, *10*(3), 102. https://doi.org/10.4103/ajm.ajm_119_20

Jonsen, A. R., Siegler, M., & Winslade, W. J. (2015). *Clinical ethics: A practical approach to ethical decisions in clinical medicine* (8th ed.). McGraw-Hill Education.

Reiner, G. (2022, October). A systematic approach to ethical decision-making for nurses [Review of *A Systematic approach to ethical decision-making for nurses*]. *Nurses Service Organization*. www.apna.org/news/a-systematic-approach-for-ethical-decision-making-for-nurses

Ulrich, C. (2012). *Nursing ethics in everyday practice*. Sigma Theta Tau International.

NCLEX FORMAT REVIEW QUESTIONS

Arrange the steps of the process of ethical decision-making in the proper order.

1. _____ Gather additional data needed.
2. _____ Make a decision.
3. _____ Clarify the existing ethical dilemma.
4. _____ Identify existing options.
5. _____ Implement actions associated with the decision.
6. _____ Evaluate decisions and the implemented actions.

Answer: 3, 1, 4, 2, 5, 6

7. A healthcare team is using Jonsen's Four Topics Method for ethical decision-making. The team is trying to determine the patient's prospects for a return to normal life with treatment. The nurse recognizes that this question is classified under:

   a. medical indications

   b. patient preferences

   c. quality of life

   d. contextual features

Answer: c

8. A healthcare team is analyzing the situation of a comatose patient who cannot provide consent regarding treatment. The team is trying to determine who is the designated surrogate to make decisions regarding the patient's treatment. Using Jonsen's Four

Topics Method for ethical decision-making, the nurse recognizes that this question is classified under:

a. medical indications
b. patient preferences
c. quality of life
d. contextual features

Answer: b

9. A healthcare team is trying to determine the goals of treatment for a patient who is comatose. Using Jonsen's Four Topics Method for ethical decision-making, the nurse recognizes that this question is classified under:

    a. medical indications
    b. patient preferences
    c. quality of life
    d. contextual features

Answer: a

10. A healthcare team is using Jonsen's Four Topics Methods to analyze the situation of a comatose patient. The team is trying to determine whether there are existing religious issues that could influence clinical decisions about the patient. The nurse recognizes that this question is classified under:

    a. medical indications
    b. patient preferences
    c. quality of life
    d. contextual features

Answer: d

TEAM-BUILDING EXERCISE

Instructions: Divide students into teams of at least three people and preferably no more than five. Each person should have a role assigned in the exercise. One person will be the leader, one person will be the timekeeper, and one person will be the recorder. The **leader** will oversee helping the discussion progress so that the objectives of the exercise are accomplished. The **timekeeper** should intervene when necessary to keep the discussion focused on the topic of the exercise and should periodically remind team members of the amount of time remaining to complete the exercise. The **recorder** will be responsible for taking notes during the discussion that can be utilized when the exercise results are presented to the class. If additional team members are included in the group, one person can be assigned to assist with the note-taking and transcription process, and the additional person can assist the team leader in guiding the discussion and assist in preparing the final presentation of the results.

SCENARIO FOR TEAM-BUILDING EXERCISE

Mr. and Mrs. Smith are members of a very strict, ultra-conservative religious community. They have one child, Mary, who has been diagnosed with a particularly virulent form of leukemia. The specialist has informed the Smiths that the cancer is treatable but that treatment must begin immediately. The Smiths are reluctant to treat Mary with anything other than holistic or herbal remedies because of their religious beliefs. The healthcare team is very concerned that Mary's condition will begin to deteriorate rapidly unless treatment is initiated quickly.

QUESTIONS

1. Identify the various ethical dilemmas that exist in this scenario.

2. Implement the process of ethical decision-making to resolve the situation.

   a. Clarify the existing ethical dilemma (see question 1).

   b. Determine the relevant stakeholders.

   c. What are the specific value conflicts that exist?

   d. What is the time frame for coming to a decision?

   e. Are there legal issues that could apply in this case?

   f. What are the viable alternatives?

   g. Select an option for the resolution of the issue.

3. Apply the three tests to determine whether the best option was selected to resolve the situation.

4. Apply Jonsen's Four Topics Method for ethical decision-making to the situation.

5. After applying both the standard method for ethical decision-making and Jonsen's Four Topics Method, which one does the team view as being most effective in generating a solution? Be able to support the answer.

6. The hospital ethics committee opts to convene to discuss Mary Smith's situation. Discuss how the committee's analysis of the case will likely proceed.

CHAPTER 4

ETHICS AND PROFESSIONAL NURSING PRACTICE

CHAPTER OBJECTIVES

After studying this chapter, students will be able to:

- Verbalize the overall purpose of the American Nurses Association *Code of Ethics for Nurses.*
- Describe ways to incorporate the provisions of the *Code of Ethics for Nurses* into modern nursing practice.
- Discuss patient advocacy and its importance as described in the *Code of Ethics for Nurses.*
- Discuss professional nursing accountability and its importance as described in the *Code of Ethics for Nurses.*
- Describe patients' rights and their importance as described in the *Code of Ethics for Nurses.*
- Discuss health promotion techniques and their importance in the *Code of Ethics for Nurses.*
- Discuss the importance of assessing the ethical environment of each nurse's workforce setting as indicated in the *Code of Ethics for Nurses.*
- Discuss ways that nurses can engage in scholarly inquiry and its importance as described in the *Code of Ethics for Nurses.*
- Discuss ways that nurses can promote social justice and its importance as described in the *Code of Ethics for Nurses.*
- Discuss global health and the global health community and what nursing can do to promote human and environmental health.

KEY TERMS

bullying
exclusion
gossip
incivility
lateral violence
social justice
verbal abuse

As discussed in the previous chapter, the modern nurse must be prepared to encounter every type of ethical dilemma, including those that have always been a concern since the nursing profession had its infancy and those that have only come into the ethical spotlight since the COVID pandemic. Thankfully, the modern nurse has the American Nurses Association *Code of Ethics for Nurses* to use as a map to guide nursing practice and help in avoiding ethical dilemmas. This chapter will discuss each provision of the *Code of Ethics for Nurses* and how each one can be interpreted to provide the most guidance to achieve the highest quality patient care outcomes.

AMERICAN NURSES ASSOCIATION *CODE OF ETHICS FOR NURSES*

- **Provision 1:** The nurse practices with compassion and respect for the inherent dignity, worth, and unique attributes of every person.
- **Provision 2:** A nurse's primary commitment is to the recipient(s) of nursing care, whether an individual, family, group, community, or population.
- **Provision 3:** The nurse establishes a trusting relationship and advocates for the rights, health, and safety of recipient(s) of nursing care.
- **Provision 4:** Nurses have authority over nursing practice and are responsible and accountable for their practice consistent with their obligations to promote health, prevent illness, and provide optimal care.
- **Provision 5:** The nurse has moral duties to self as a person of inherent dignity and worth including an expectation of a safe place to work that fosters flourishing, authenticity of self at work, and self-respect through integrity and professional competence.
- **Provision 6:** Nurses, through individual and collective effort, establish, maintain, and improve the ethical environment of the work setting that affects nursing care and the well-being of nurses.

- **Provision 7:** Nurses advance the profession through multiple approaches to knowledge development, professional standards, and the generation of policies for nursing, health, and social concerns.
- **Provision 8:** Nurses build collaborative relationships and networks with nurses, other healthcare and non-healthcare disciplines, and the public to achieve greater ends.
- **Provision 9:** The profession of nursing, collectively through its professional organizations, must articulate nursing values, maintain the integrity of the profession, and integrate principles of social justice into nursing and health policy.
- **Provision 10:** Nursing, through organizations and associations, participates in the global nursing and health community to promote human and environmental health, well-being, and flourishing.[1]

Provision 1

Provision 1 of the code addresses the importance of the nurse demonstrating compassion in his or her nursing practice, as well as respect for the worth of the individual. How can compassion be defined in terms of nursing care of the patient? Su et al. (2021) indicated that *compassion* refers to the nurse's sensitivity toward the suffering of others and a desire to alleviate such misery. It is viewed as a central tenet of the nursing profession, as shown by Watson's Human Caring Theory. Compassionate care has been linked to improved patient care outcomes during hospitalization and tends to lead to improved patient compliance with treatment regimens. Aagard et al. (2018) indicated in an international research study that *compassion* is defined as demonstrating caring along with listening, developing a relationship with patients and the members of their support systems, making an effort to alleviate suffering, connecting with the patient empathetically, and ultimately going beyond what would usually be expected in the nurse's role. The American Association of Colleges of Nursing (2025a) noted that nurses who demonstrate compassionate care in nursing practice exhibit the following characteristics:

- Integrity—the nurse's behavior is congruent with his or her expressed values
- Excellence—the nurse has obvious clinical expertise

1. American Nurses Association, Selection from "Contents," *Code of Ethics for Nurses*, pp. vii–ix. Copyright © 2022 by American Nurses Association.

- Compassion—the nurse is aware of the patient's suffering and seeks to relieve it
- Altruism—the nurse puts the needs of the patient before the nurse's own needs
- Respect—the nurse recognizes the values as well as the autonomy of the patient
- Empathy—the nurse is able to put himself or herself in the patient's situation
- Service—the nurse goes beyond what is required to share time and resources

As previously mentioned, part of this provision includes the importance of the nurse respecting the worth of the individual. According to the American Association of Colleges of Nursing (2025b) this can be accomplished through the nurse identifying the needs and values of the patient. This will allow patient care to be individualized to accommodate what the patient considers to be a priority, whether it is the need for a specialized diet because of religious beliefs or the need for breakthrough pain relief because of a terminal illness. It is the responsibility of the nurse to set aside his or her innate biases so that the nurse–patient relationship can develop through a gradual increase in trust. This can occur only if the nurse respects the decisions of the patient even if the nurse doesn't necessarily agree with those decisions. The nurse also demonstrates respect for the patient's worth as an individual by making certain that the patient receives the highest quality patient care possible, regardless of the patient's type of illness or socioeconomic resources available. This can take place as the nurse ensures that the patient and his or her support system have all the information needed to make a fully informed decision regarding a choice of medical treatments, medications, and specialists. Finally, the nurse will demonstrate respect for the worth of the patient through the development of teamwork with colleagues on the patient's healthcare team. This will increase the likelihood that the patient's healthcare goals will be achieved.

Provision 2

The main commitment of the nurse must always be to the recipient of care, and therefore the nurse may serve as an advocate for the patient as well as members of his or her support system and the overall community.

What does it mean to act as a patient advocate? Nsiah et al. (2019) found that nurses described patient advocacy as:

> Protecting the patient—the nurse recognizes that the patient has a certain degree of vulnerability, particularly in a clinical setting. The nurse acts as a patient advocate by defending his or her rights when needed and protecting the patient from not only injuries that may occur but also any action by family members or members of the healthcare team that could impede the patient's recovery.
>
> Serving as the patient's voice—the nurse recognizes the importance of speaking for the patient to express his or her needs and preferences if the patient is unable to speak. The nurse also makes certain that the patient's wishes are paramount in the process of care collaboration even if they conflict with those of family members.
>
> Providing quality care—what exemplifies quality nursing care? Quality nursing care ideally leads to the achievement of high-quality patient care outcomes. According to the World Health Organization (2025), hallmarks of quality healthcare include the following attributes:

- effective—the nurse provides care to whoever is in need, whether it is the patient, his or her family members, or the surrounding community.
- safe—the nurse avoids harm coming to the recipients of care.
- people-centered—the nurse collaborates with the patient and healthcare team in developing a plan of care that incorporates the patient's preferences, needs, and values.
- timely—the nurse does everything possible to avoid delays in care that could be harmful to the patient.
- equitable—the nurse ensures that the care that he or she provides does not vary regardless of the patient's gender, ethnicity, geographic location, socioeconomic status, or similar factors.
- integrated—the care provided by the nurse incorporates all health services that may be available throughout the course of the patient's life.
- efficient—the nurse recognizes the importance of conserving available resources in terms of healthcare supplies and staffing hours, for example.

Developing an interpersonal nurse-patient relationship—the nurse recognizes the necessity of encouraging trust to develop between the nurse and the patient as they collaborate on the plan of care. Trust will develop in the relationship as the patient feels valued by the nurse, begins to feel comfortable with expressing his or her thoughts and preferences regarding treatment, and both the patient and nurse feel a mutual respect. Trust can develop as the nurse practices therapeutic communication techniques as he or she works with the patient. According to the *American Nurse Journal* (2025), there are several techniques that the nurse can incorporate to assist in developing the nurse-patient relationship. These include the following:

- using silence—use of intentional silence can give both patient and nurse the opportunity to process what has already been discussed. The patient may be overwhelmed by the sheer volume of information that they have been given regarding their situation. Allow the patient to break the silence as an indicator that he or she is prepared to move on to another topic.
- accepting—this is acknowledgment that the nurse has heard what the patient is saying. It is not synonymous with agreement, but it does indicate to the patient that the nurse takes them seriously.
- giving recognition—this is not a compliment, but it does draw attention to a patient's behavior that is positive and encourages it to continue.
- offering self—simply taking the time to stay and talk with patients for a few minutes can be indicative of the value that the nurse places on the relationship.
- giving broad openings—this allows the patient to direct the conversational flow. It will indicate to the nurse what is most important to the patient.
- active listening—use both verbal and nonverbal cues to encourage patients to continue the conversation. Show interest in the patient's discussion and stay engaged throughout the conversation.
- seeking clarification—ask patients for more information if they have said something confusing to ensure that the nurse clearly understands the trend of the conversation.

- placing the event in time or sequence—ask questions about when specific events occurred in relation to other events so that both patient and nurse can gain a clarified view of the sequence.
- making observations—if the nurse makes an observation regarding the patient's appearance or behavior, for example, it may prompt the patient to provide new information about recent symptoms.
- encouraging descriptions of perception—if the patient is experiencing some type of sensory issue, it may help them to express themselves more succinctly if the nurse encourages the patient to describe what he or she is seeing or hearing.
- encouraging comparisons—this allows the patient to draw upon past experience to deal with the current problem.
- summarizing—this shows the patient that the nurse was listening and allows the nurse to document the conversation accurately.
- reflecting—if the nurse asks the patient what he or she thinks they should do about a specific problem, the patient is more likely to develop a solution without additional guidance. This also encourages patients to be accountable for their own actions.
- focusing—if the patient mentions something that is of particular importance, the nurse can focus on this statement and encourage the patient to discuss it in additional detail.
- confronting—this should only be used once trust has been established. It may be essential to use confrontation to help patients break a behavior pattern that can be detrimental to their health.
- voicing doubt—this is intended to gently call attention to an incorrect idea or perception of a patient so that it can be reexamined.
- offering hope and humor—lightening the mood can be a stress reliever for patients and can help nurse-patient rapport develop rapidly. It may help keep the patient's mindset more positive and may strengthen the bond of trust between patient and nurse.

TABLE 4.1 TECHNIQUES TO HELP DEVELOP THE NURSE-PATIENT RELATIONSHIP

Using silence	use of intentional silence gives patient and nurse the opportunity to process what has already been discussed
Accepting	acknowledgment that the nurse has heard what the patient is saying; indicates that the nurse takes the patient seriously
Giving recognition	draws attention to patient's behavior that is positive and encourages it to continue
Offering self	taking the time to stay and talk with patients for a few minutes indicates the value that the nurse places on the relationship
Giving broad openings	allows the patient to direct the conversational flow; indicates to the nurse what is most important to the patient
Active listening	use both verbal and nonverbal cues to encourage patients to continue the conversation
Seeking clarification	ask patients for more information if they have said something confusing
Placing the event in time or sequence	ask questions about when specific events occurred in relation to other events
Making observations	nurse makes an observation about patient's appearance or behavior
Encouraging description of perceptions	may help the patients who are experiencing some type of sensory issue to express themselves more effectively
Encouraging comparisons	allows patient to draw upon past experience to deal with the current problem
Summarizing	shows patient that the nurse was listening and also allows the nurse to document the conversation accurately
Reflecting	the nurse asks the patient what he or she thinks should be done about a specific problem, thus allowing the patient to develop a solution without additional guidance
Focusing	if the patient mentions something that is of particular importance, the nurse can focus on this statement and encourage the patient to discuss it in additional detail
Confronting	this should only be used once trust has been established
Voicing doubt	call attention to an incorrect idea or perception of a patient so that it can be reexamined
Offering hope and humor	lighten the mood to relieve stress and develop rapport

Provision 3

The nurse is responsible for promoting, advocating for, and protecting the patient's rights, health, and safety. Patient advocacy has been previously discussed, but how can the nurse successfully protect the patient's rights? According to the National Institutes of Health Clinical Center (2025), patient rights include the right:

- to be cared for in a safe, considerate, and respectful manner that is congruent with the patient's belief system; this requires the nurse to maintain the role of advocate in ensuring that all members of the healthcare team take the time and effort needed to verify the patient's beliefs.
- to expect that all patient records will be considered confidential in accordance with HIPAA requirements; this requires the nurse to stay up-to-date on all training related to HIPAA, privacy, and confidentiality requirements.
- to know the physician responsible for coordinating the patient's care; this may also require the nurse to act as patient advocate to ensure that the patient recognizes that he or she is the most important member of the healthcare team.
- to receive complete information regarding the diagnosis, treatment, and prognosis in layman's terms; if the patient clearly does not have a full understanding of his or her illness and treatment plan, the nurse is responsible for contacting the healthcare provider to arrange for the provider or designee to talk with the patient regarding this.
- to receive sufficient information to allow the patient to provide informed consent before any procedure or treatment; if the patient does not have sufficient information to legally provide informed consent, the nurse is responsible for contacting the healthcare provider to make certain that the procedure does not progress until such information is provided to the patient.
- to have pain accurately assessed and treated appropriately; as the pioneer pain management expert Margo McCaffery noted, pain is whatever the patient experiencing it says it is and thus requires the nurse to be vigilant in assessing the patient at frequent intervals for obvious symptoms of pain, as well as evidence of stoicism (Cox, 2022).
- to refuse treatment and to be informed of the potential medical consequences of such refusal; this situation may require the ultimate nurse advocate, since the nurse may have to protect the patient's right to end treatment and potentially progress toward a

death of his or her choosing amid the opposition of the patient's family members and other members of the healthcare team.

This is by no means intended to be an exhaustive list of all possible patient rights. More specific examples of patient rights can be found in specialized facilities.

TABLE 4.2 PATIENT'S RIGHTS

to be cared for in a safe, considerate, and respectful manner that is congruent with the patient's belief system	requires the nurse to serve as advocate in ensuring that all members of the healthcare team verify patient's beliefs
to expect that all patient records will be considered confidential in accordance with HIPAA requirements	the nurse stays up-to-date on all training related to HIPAA, privacy, and confidentiality requirements
to know the physician responsible for coordinating the patient's care	the nurse acts as patient advocate so that the patient recognizes that he or she is the most important member of the team
to receive complete information regarding the diagnosis, treatment, and prognosis in layman's terms	if the patient does not understand illness/treatment plan, the nurse must contact the provider
to receive sufficient information to allow the patient to provide informed consent before any procedure or treatment	if the patient does not have sufficient information to provide informed consent, the nurse contacts provider so that the procedure does not progress until information is provided
to have pain accurately assessed and treated appropriately	nurse must assess patient for symptoms of pain as well as evidence of stoicism
to refuse treatment and to be informed of the potential medical consequences of such refusal	the nurse protects patient's right to end treatment and progress toward death

Provision 4

The nurse has authority over nursing practice and is both responsible and accountable for his or her practice. A nurse's practice should be consistent with his or her obligations to promote health as well as prevent illness and provide optimal patient care. The nurse also commits to use his or her talent and energy to improve patient outcomes. Nurses are expected to take ownership of their actions and therefore must hold themselves accountable not only individually but also as members of a healthcare team.

Sherman and Cohn (2019) noted that professional nursing accountability includes the following:

- functioning within the nursing scope of practice as defined by each state's Board of Nursing
- complying with professional standards through educational updates as the standards are revised
- providing patient care utilizing evidence-based practice
- sharing accountability with other members of the healthcare team to generate high-quality patient care outcomes
- following documented workplace policies and procedures

Ideally, the nurse is accountable for his or her actions and consequently functions in accordance with professional standards not merely because the nurse is required to do so by the profession or by the facility, but because the nurse expects it of himself or herself.

Provision 5

The nurse is obligated to provide the same duties to self as to others, including promoting health and safety, preserving character and integrity, maintaining competence, and continuing to pursue personal and professional growth. Adequate self-care in nurses may help them avoid burnout and consequently remain in the profession longer. Couser et al. (2020) noted that nurses frequently tend to neglect their own self-care needs as they devote their time to patient care. The American Nurses Association (2017) indicated that 82% of nurses reported feeling that they were at significant risk of developing workplace stress. To combat this, nurses should be encouraged to practice the same health promotion techniques that they use in patient education sessions. These include the following:

- regular exercise to assist in achieving weight control, improved heart health, and increased muscle strength
- developing a sleep routine that will allow for quality sleep
- practicing adequate nutrition and hydration, particularly adding high-protein, high-fiber foods to a regular diet
- selecting and pursuing a hobby to achieve a more effective life-work balance
- practicing self-reflection to achieve greater self-understanding and to recognize emotions being experienced
- seeking support from colleagues as well as members of the support system—developing a support network can reduce

feelings of isolation and loneliness. Sharing experiences with other nurses can allow collegial connections to develop and reduce the experience of employment-related frustration. As a nurse develops his or her support network, the consequent feelings of being nurtured will help reduce the impulse to ignore the nurse's own needs for self-care.

- setting boundaries—when the nurse feels confident enough to refuse additional shifts when he or she is already exhausted, the nurse sets the stage to become a more effective worker who is more patient and compassionate and also capable of greater critical thinking due to being well-rested (Couser et al., 2020).

Provision 6

The nurse is responsible, both individually and as a member of the healthcare team, for maintaining and improving the ethical environment of the work setting. How can a nurse assess the ethical environment of his or her professional setting? The American Nurses Association (2021) recommends the use of tools such as

- the Hospital Ethical Climate Survey,
- the Moral Distress Thermometer,
- the Measure of Moral Distress in Health Care Professionals,
- the American Association of Critical-Care Nurses Healthy Work Environment Assessment Tool, and
- the National League for Nursing's revised Healthful Work Environment Toolkit.

Workplace environments that are assessed and found to be characterized by incivility, bullying, and lateral violence are considered to be not only unethical but also high risk for damage to patient safety and the professional integrity of healthcare team members. Alsadaan et al. (2024) has described **incivility** as disrespectful behavior toward nurses that may be overt or covert. **Bullying** and **verbal abuse** are categorized as overt forms of incivility, while **gossip** and **exclusion** are considered to be examples of its covert form. When harassment behavior occurs between coworkers who have essentially equal status, the incivility is labeled as **lateral violence**. Vidal-Alves et al. (2021) noted that lateral violence among nurses is strongly correlated with higher levels of burnout, decreased job satisfaction, and poor health indicators, all of which can increase rates of nurse turnover.

How can the incidence of lateral violence be decreased once the ethical environment of a facility has been assessed? According to Rainford et al. (2015), the facility must undergo a cultural shift, particularly when the organization has been inadvertently ignoring or even fostering such behavior. Lateral violence is especially prevalent in facilities where nurses are undervalued and are working with unrealistic patient assignments while trying to complete multiple critical tasks. As facilities struggle to cope with continued nursing shortages, budget cuts, program restructuring, and changing healthcare regulations, lateral violence in the healthcare workforce is likely to persist.

Provision 7

The nurse is responsible for advancing the profession through development of knowledge, and consequently of professional standards, and the creation of both nursing and health policy. How can nurses participate in scholarly inquiry that may lay the foundation for new health policy? Rocel and Williams (2024) note that the Magnet Recognition Program can be used to help nurses visualize the relationship between scholarly research, nursing practice, and high-quality patient outcomes. The Magnet Recognition Program places emphasis on promoting quality in a healthcare setting that is supportive of professional practice and recognizes outstanding nursing care while also disseminating best practices in nursing. In addition, the program emphasizes helping nurses influence any aspect of the healthcare organization that impacts nursing practice, including both the development of patient outcomes and the practice environment being utilized. One specific component of the Magnet Recognition Program encourages healthcare organizations to be supportive of nurses as they pursue scholarly work by providing education and resources that will expedite the research and incorporating evidence-based practice into nursing care.

To promote the incorporation of nursing research into daily nursing practice, Rocel and Williams (2024) provide some suggestions that will help encourage nurses to review and critique research studies and potentially incorporate them into clinical practice. These include the following:

- implement a research journal committee that meets regularly to both review and critique research articles; encourage nursing staff to suggest research possibilities and also to critically appraise current research initiatives
- emphasize the importance of evidence-based nursing practice in schools of nursing; this sets the stage for the rising generation

of nurses to already have the importance of nursing research incorporated into their professional psyches

- encourage attendance at research presentations; participation in poster presentations is an easy way for nurses to incorporate evidence-based research findings into clinical practice and sets the stage for nurses to further springboard into more extensive research
- encourage nurses to serve as coinvestigators in research projects to increase nurses' knowledge of the research process
- offer continuing education offerings so that nurses can frequently review the research process and consequently become more proficient at implementing it
- ensure that research findings are actually incorporated into nursing practice to reinforce the importance of implementing the research process

Provision 8

The nurse is responsible for collaborating with other health professionals, the public, and governmental entities to protect human rights, promote global health, and reduce health disparities. According to the U.S. Centers for Disease Control and Prevention (2024), health disparities are preventable differences in populations related to disease, injury, violence, or opportunities. A population that experiences limited access to the resources needed to be healthy will be more likely to experience health issues. Consequently, healthcare delivery can inadvertently be linked to unequal health outcomes that are related to race and ethnicity. The patient's perception of discrimination can lead to a delay in seeking out a healthcare provider, thus increasing the likelihood of a decreased health outcome. The American Nurses Association (2025) has indicated that civility should be implemented to enhance mutual respect and promote communication as well as collaboration between nurses, other members of the healthcare team, and above all, the patient.

The American Nurses Association recommends the following activities be implemented to be as inclusive as possible in practice settings, policy creation, and advocacy:

- nurses must recognize discriminatory practices so that they can be addressed
- nurses must be capable of self-reflection regarding their personal and professional values so that potential conflicts can be resolved in the best interest of the patient

- nurses should support nursing practice environments that embrace inclusivity and promote civility and respect regarding patients, members of the healthcare team, and the community
- nurses should incorporate the concepts of justice, caring, diversity, inclusiveness, civility, and mutual respect as guiding principles that they utilize as they provide healthcare
- nurses should support and implement research that is inclusive and includes the healthcare needs of diverse populations
- nurse managers, supervisors, and administrators must assess policies for evidence of inclusiveness, civility, and mutual respect
- nurse educators must promote a diverse workforce by developing practices in academia that will both attract and retain students from all backgrounds
- nurses must incorporate a patient-centered approach in response to the cultural concerns of patients and their support systems

Provision 9

The profession of nursing is responsible for promoting nursing values, maintaining the integrity of the profession, and integrating the principles of social justice. How can nurses promote social justice? The American Association of Colleges of Nursing has described **social justice** as providing fair treatment for all individuals regardless of the patient's economic status, race, ethnicity, age, sexual orientation, citizenship, or disability (Habibzadeh, 2021). To promote this positive concept, the American Nurses Association (2020) has encouraged nurses to remove areas of bias in nursing practice that continue to reinforce negative behaviors and stereotypes. Nurses should collaborate with other members of the healthcare team, policy makers, and leaders in the healthcare industry to address identified negative behaviors that can lead to specific individuals and communities failing to receive the healthcare treatment that they should receive. Nurses' role as change agent can be invaluable as they work within their own healthcare facilities to make the institutions more inclusive and more free of bias, whether overt or less obvious. In addition, nurses' role as advocate can further the development of policies at the local facility level, as well as the state and national levels, that will address the need to ensure health equity for all individuals. Such policies will improve the provision of healthcare and ensure more positive patient care outcomes. Once nurses are committed to identifying and eliminating areas of bias in healthcare, the foundation is laid for the creation and maintenance of a culture of inclusion within the profession and in the healthcare community (American Nurses Association, 2020).

Provision 10

Nurses must participate in the global nursing and health community in an effort to promote both human health and environmental health. Global health issues are multifaceted and complex and are increasing in number, as shown by the repercussions from the recent pandemic and the pressure on healthcare consumers to be vaccinated against each annual variant of the COVID virus. Global health concerns include not only issues such as infectious diseases and maternal mortality but also issues such as human trafficking, immigration, and racism. How can nurses contribute to the resolution of such concerns? Initially, nurses must educate themselves on global health issues, the issues' significance to healthcare, and the impact on patient populations. Once nurses have a clear understanding of the various facets of an issue, the stage is set for nurses to move forward into a leadership role and exert influence. The nurse leaders of today who will move into the next decades must exercise a high level of innovation and creativity that is balanced with an equally high level of critical thinking. Only when the nurse leader is able to be a role model for other nurses through being both visionary and a change agent can change occur that will be sustained (Edmonson et al., 2017).

In summary, the *Code of Ethics for Nurses* should be utilized as an invaluable guidebook as nurse leaders try to promote high-quality patient care outcomes in a rapidly changing healthcare environment. In subsequent chapters, the use of the *Code of Ethics for Nurses* will be discussed in connection with specific patient populations.

REFERENCES

Aagard, M., Papadopoulos, I., & Biles, J. (January 26, 2018). Exploring compassion in U.S. nurses: Results from an international research study. *OJIN: The Online Journal of Issues in Nursing, 23*(1). https://doi.org/10.3912/OJIN.Vol23No01PPT44

Alsadaan, N., Ramadan, O.M.E., & Alqahtani, M. (2024). From incivility to outcomes: Tracing the effects of nursing incivility on nurse well-being, patient engagement, and health outcomes. *BMC Nursing, 23*(325). https://doi.org/10.1186/s12912-024-01996-9

American Association of Colleges of Nursing. (2025a). Compassionate care. 5B Toolkit. Retrieved from https://www.aacnnursing.org/5b-tool-kit/themes/compassionate-care.

American Association of Colleges of Nursing (2025b). Respect. 5B Toolkit. Retrieved from https://www.aacnnursing.org/5b-tool-kit/themes/respect.

American Nurses Association. (2017). *Executive summary, American Nurses Association health risk appraisal.* https://www.nursingworld.org/~495c56/globalassets/practice-andpolicy/healthy-nurse-healthy-nation/ana-healthriskappraisalsummary_2013-2016.pdf.

American Nurses Association. (2020). *The American Academy of Nursing and the American Nurses Association call for social justice to address racism and health equity in communities of color.* https://www.nursingworld.org/news/news-releases/2020/the-american-academy-of-nursing-and-the-american-nurses-association-call-for-social-justice-to-address-racism-and-health-equity-in-communities-of-color/.

American Nurses Association. (2021). *Nurses' professional responsibility to promote ethical practice environments.* https://www.nursingworld.org/globalassets/practiceandpolicy/nursing-excellence/ana-position-statements/nursing-practice/nurses-professional-responsibility-to-promote-ethical-practice-environments-2021-final.pdf.

American Nurses Association. (2025). Code of ethics with interpretative statements. https://codeofethics.ana.org/home#.

American Nurse Journal. (2025). What is therapeutic communication? https://www.myamericannurse.com/therapeutic-communication-techniques/.

ANA Ethics Advisory Board. (2019, June 7). ANA position statement: The nurse's role in addressing discrimination: Protecting and promoting inclusive strategies in practice settings, policy, and advocacy. *OJIN: The Online Journal of Issues in Nursing, 24*(3).

Couser, G., Chesak, S., & Cutshall, S. (2020, August 14). Developing a course to promote self-care for nurses to address burnout. *OJIN: The Online Journal of Issues in Nursing, 25*(3).

Cox, F. (2022, March 30). An overview of pain assessment and management. Nursing Standard. Advance online publication. https://doi.org/10.7748/ns.2022.e11936

Edmonson, C., McCarthy, C., Trent-Adams, S., McCain, C., & Marshall, J. (2017, January 31). Emerging global health issues: A nurse's role. *OJIN: The Online Journal of Issues in Nursing, 22*(1), Manuscript 2.

Habibzadeh, H., Jasemi, M., & Hosseinzadegan, F. (2021). Social justice in health system; a neglected component of academic nursing education: A qualitative study. *BMC Nursing, 20*(16). https://doi.org/10.1186/s12912-021-00534-1.

National Institutes of Health Clinical Center. (2025). Patient bill of rights. https://www.cc.nih.gov/patient-info/legal/bill-of-rights.

Nsiah, C., Siakwa, M., & Ninnoni, J. P. K. (2019, May 29). Registered Nurses' description of patient advocacy in the clinical setting. *Nursing Open, 6*(3), 1124–1132. https://doi.org/10.1002/nop2.307

Rainford, W., Wood, S., McMullen, P., & Philipsen, N. (2015). The disruptive force of lateral violence in the health care setting. *The Journal for Nurse Practitioners, 11*(2), 157–164. https://doi.org/10.1016/j.nurpra.2014.10.010.

Rocel, B., & Williams, D. (2024). Engaging nurses in scholarly work. *American Nurse Journal, 19*(1), 50–56. https://doi.org/10.51256/anj012450

Sherman, R., & Cohn, T. (2019, February). Promoting professional accountability and ownership [Review of *Promoting professional accountability and ownership*]. *American Nurse Today, 14*(2), 24–26. https://www.myamericannurse.com/wp-content/uploads/2019/02/ant2-Accountability-117.pdf

Su, J. J., Paguio, J. T., Masika, G. M., Wang, M., & Redding, S. R. (2021). Learning compassionate care: Experiences of nursing students. *Nurse Education in Practice*, *53*(103092), 103092. https://doi.org/10.1016/j.nepr.2021.103092

U.S. Centers for Disease Control and Prevention. (2024). What is health equity? Retrieved from https://www.cdc.gov/health-equity/what-is/index.html.

Vidal-Alves, M. J., Pina, D., Puente-López, E., Luna-Maldonado, A., Luna Ruiz-Cabello, A., Magalhães, T., Pina-López, Y., Ruiz-Hernández, J. A., & Jarreta, B. M. (2021). Tough Love Lessons: Lateral Violence among Hospital Nurses. *International Journal of Environmental Research and Public Health*, 18(17), 9183. https://doi.org/10.3390/ijerph18179183

World Health Organization. (2025). Quality of care. Retrieved from https://www.who.int/health-topics/quality-of-care#tab=tab_1.

NCLEX FORMAT REVIEW QUESTIONS

Match the provision number with its basic premise.

1. Provision 1 ____
2. Provision 2 ____
3. Provision 3 ____
4. Provision 4 ____
5. Provision 5 ____
6. Provision 6 ____
7. Provision 7 ____
8. Provision 8 ____
9. Provision 9 ____
10. Provision 10 ____

a. the nurse advances the profession through research and scholarly inquiry

b. the nurse owes the same duties to self as to others

c. the nurse maintains and improves the ethical environment of the work setting

d. the nurse advocates for and protects the rights, health, and safety of the patient

e. the nurse has authority, accountability, and responsibility for nursing practice

f. the nurse collaborates with other health professionals and the public

g. the nurse's primary commitment is to the patient

h. the profession of nursing must integrate principles of social justice into nursing

i. the nurse practices with compassion and respect for the dignity of every person

j. the nurse participates in the global nursing community to promote health

Answers:

1. i	4. e	7. a	10. j
2. g	5. b	8. f	
3. d	6. c	9. h	

TEAM-BUILDING EXERCISE

Instructions: Divide students into teams of at least three people and preferably no more than five. Each person should have a role assigned in the exercise. One person will be the leader, one person will be the timekeeper, and one person will be the recorder. The **leader** will oversee helping the discussion progress so that the objectives of the exercise are accomplished. The **timekeeper** should intervene when necessary to keep the discussion focused on the topic of the exercise and should periodically remind team members of the amount of time remaining to complete the exercise. The **recorder** will be responsible for taking notes during the discussion that can be utilized when the exercise results are presented to the class. If additional team members are included in the group, one person can be assigned to assist with the note-taking and transcription process, and the additional person can assist the team leader in guiding the discussion and assist in preparing the final presentation of the results.

SCENARIO FOR TEAM-BUILDING EXERCISE

Joe is the daytime charge nurse on a 40-bed medical oncology floor. The floor is not fully staffed, having a total of six vacant positions open between both shifts. All the nurses including Joe are working overtime. The floor is a particularly stressful one to work on because of the volatile nature of one of the oncologists, Dr. Smith. Although Joe has a working relationship with Dr. Smith, the oncologist engages in frequent shouting matches with some nurses and leaves others in tears. Joe would like to cut back on his work hours so that he can go back to school for a graduate degree but is hesitant to leave his staff without a buffer to "run interference" between them and Dr. Smith.

QUESTIONS

1. Analyze the scenario and decide how provision 1 of the *Code of Ethics for Nurses* would be applicable in this case.

2. Analyze the scenario and decide how provision 2 of the *Code of Ethics for Nurses* would be applicable in this case.

3. Analyze the scenario and decide how provision 3 of the *Code of Ethics for Nurses* would be applicable in this case.

4. Analyze the scenario and decide how provision 4 of the *Code of Ethics for Nurses* would be applicable in this case.

5. Analyze the scenario and decide how provision 5 of the *Code of Ethics for Nurses* would be applicable in this case.

6. Analyze the scenario and decide how provision 6 of the *Code of Ethics for Nurses* would be applicable in this case.

7. Analyze the scenario and decide how provision 7 of the *Code of Ethics for Nurses* would be applicable in this case.

8. Analyze the scenario and decide how provision 8 of the *Code of Ethics for Nurses* would be applicable in this case.

9. Analyze the scenario and decide how provision 9 of the *Code of Ethics for Nurses* would be applicable in this case.

10. Analyze the scenario and decide how provision 10 of the *Code of Ethics for Nurses* would be applicable in this case.

CHAPTER 5

ETHICAL ISSUES PERTAINING TO CHILDREN AND ADOLESCENTS

CHAPTER OBJECTIVES

After studying this chapter, students will be able to:

- Discuss the important ethical questions that will arise in pediatric healthcare.
- Discuss the ethical concerns that may arise for nurses caring for critically ill children.
- Compare and contrast the ethical issues that may arise for critically ill children and for adolescent patients.
- Describe the status of the emancipated minor.
- Discuss the exceptions to the standard procedure of obtaining parental or legal guardian content to provide medical treatment to a minor.
- Describe the difference between a patient assenting to treatment and providing a consent to treatment.
- Analyze the three essential elements of informed consent as they apply to the adolescent patient.
- Discuss the limits of confidentiality as they apply to the adolescent patient.
- Describe how a nurse can develop ethical numbness.
- Discuss how a pediatric nurse could develop moral distress.
- Describe the strategies that could assist the pediatric nurse in developing resilience.
- Analyze the concept of moral courage and discuss how it can be developed in the pediatric nurse.

KEY TERMS

assent to treatment
consent to treatment
emancipated minor
ethical numbness
limits of confidentiality
moral courage
moral distress
resilience

Pediatric nursing is a specialty with its own unique set of ethical challenges. Carnevale (2012) noted that important ethical questions that will arise in pediatric healthcare include the following: How should healthcare decisions for children be made? and Who are the appropriate parties to make these decisions? The adults who make decisions involving a child's medical treatment must make the child's best interests paramount in their decision-making process. Their views on the importance of quality of life and what truly constitutes the child's best interest must be clearly established. It is important to determine that what constitutes the best interest of the child is not discounted to accommodate the best interests of others.

CARING FOR CRITICALLY ILL CHILDREN

The pediatric nurse who consistently cares for very critically ill children may find himself or herself frequently experiencing an ethical dilemma. The nurse's commitment to promoting the highest possible quality of life for a patient may conflict with the parents' or guardians' desire to relieve the suffering of a chronically ill child. The nurse may experience frustration and guilt if the goals of the child's family members seem to conflict with the healthcare team's established treatment plan. Emotional distress and ethical concerns may be experienced by a nurse who must administer uncomfortable treatments such as chemotherapy to a critically ill child who is already suffering from cancer and has a dwindling prognosis to recover. The nurse may question the decision to administer such treatments if they are being viewed as futile by either the team members or the child's parents. In addition, nurses caring for this population of patients report experiencing ethical concerns regarding the inability to spend extended periods of time with critically ill pediatric patients, particularly when there is clearly a need for the child to express his or her concerns related to the dying process (Furingsten et al., 2015). To minimize the possibility of conflicts occurring that will take the focus away from the provision of care to make the child's dying process as peaceful and comfortable as possible, nurses should ensure that parents or legal guardians are closely involved in the decision-making process with the healthcare team. Nurses can minimize ethical dilemmas from occurring by recognizing that a perceived failure on the part of family members to be as involved in the dying child's end-of-life care as much as the healthcare team would prefer may in fact be related to a cultural aspect that the team is unaware of (Butts & Rich, 2020).

ADOLESCENT PATIENT POPULATIONS

Nursing care of adolescent patient populations carries with it other unique ethical challenges, one of which is the status of an **emancipated minor**. According to Davis and Fang (2023), this means that the adolescent is free from parental or legal guardian control and therefore can legally consent to or refuse medical care without the need for the healthcare team to consult parents or guardians. Generally, the status of emancipated minor encompasses minors who are married, who are active-duty military, or who manage their own finances independent of a parent or legal guardian.

Emergency medical care is another exception to the standard procedure of obtaining parental or legal guardian consent to provide medical treatment to a minor. Federal law mandates under the Emergency Medical Treatment and Labor Act (EMTALA) that a medical screening exam must be performed on anyone, including minors, who arrives at a federally funded emergency department requesting treatment, regardless of whether consent has been obtained or there is ability to pay for the care provided. Once the exam is performed, if no emergency medical condition exists in the minor patient, the exception to consent no longer applies, and the parent or guardian must be contacted for consent for treatment (Davis & Fang, 2023).

De Jesus et al. (2022) emphasize the importance of distinguishing between an adolescent patient assenting to treatment and actually giving informed consent. **Assent to treatment** means that the patient is willing to accept the treatment offered by the healthcare team. In comparison, **consent to treatment** means that the patient has a capacity to make decisions about the intervention that's being proposed. Informed consent can only be given by a patient who is both competent to make a decision about treatment once sufficient information about the procedure has been provided and of legal age. Although most minor patients will not be able to legally give consent, they should be involved as much as possible in making decisions regarding treatment. According to the

American Academy of Child and Adolescent Psychiatry Code of Ethics, the healthcare team should seek assent from a minor before beginning treatment even though actual consent will be given by the parent or legal guardian. Ulrich (2012) described the three essential elements of informed consent:

- Capacity to make decisions—the adolescent must have the ability to understand the situation and the information that's presented, must be able to reason through the various alternatives that are being presented, and must be able to clearly indicate the choices that are the patient's preference
- Reasons for treatment—the adolescent must be able to understand the diagnosis, the tests that are needed to help the healthcare team understand the prognosis as well as disease progression, and the treatment options that are available
- Treatment options—the adolescent must be able to understand the risks as well as the benefits of the treatments being offered, along with the likely result of no treatments being utilized

TABLE 5.1 ESSENTIAL ELEMENT OF INFORMED CONSENT

Element	Description
Capacity to make decisions	the adolescent must have ability to understand the situation and information that's presented, must be able to reason through alternatives that are being presented, and must be able to indicate choices that are the patient's preference
Reasons for treatment	the adolescent must be able to understand the diagnosis, tests that are needed to help healthcare team understand the prognosis as well as disease progression, and treatment options available
Treatment options	the adolescent must be able to understand risks as well as benefits of treatments being offered, along with likely result of no treatments being utilized

Once the nurse begins to develop a trusting relationship with an adolescent patient, the nurse must be able to assure the patient of the confidentiality of information that the patient has provided to the nurse in confidence. The adolescent patient who feels comfortable with his or her healthcare provider may disclose valuable information that may alert team members to the presence of an abusive situation or even the presence of human trafficking. However, the nurse should recognize that confidentiality should not be guaranteed when there is a situation that places the adolescent in harm's way. This is considered to be the **limits of confidentiality** (Butts & Rich, 2020).

Choe et al. (2017) indicated that nurses practicing under highly stressful conditions can experience **ethical numbness**, particularly when there are multiple tasks to be completed in a short period of time such as occurs with a heavy nursing workload. During such a time, nurses may fail to see pediatric patients as individuals with specific needs. They may fail to follow approved protocol in order to complete as many tasks as possible. Choe et al.'s study found that ethical numbness can lead to ethical failures in nursing practice, such as inappropriately delegating treatments to family members, failing to accurately evaluate a child's pain level, and restraining a child unnecessarily.

MORAL DISTRESS

Carnevale (2012) elaborates that persistent workplace stress may contribute to pediatric nurses experiencing **moral distress**; this would occur when circumstances prevent the nurse from doing what he or she knows to be the right thing to do in a specific situation. The nurse may be caught between the needs of the child, the wishes of parents or other family members, and the treatment plan of the healthcare team, while feeling that there are no morally good alternatives and only unacceptable options. When the nurse is faced with supporting a family who must make the decision to withdraw life support from a child, there may consequently be a feeling of regret and guilt. It is important that the nurse be reassured that experiencing moral distress is simply evidence that the nurse has a sensitive human conscience and is practicing under ethically difficult conditions.

Dos Santos et al. (2018) discussed specific causes of moral distress that could potentially arise in pediatric nursing, as well as for those in other specialties:

- Providing treatment that the nurse views as being unnecessary or futile
- Providing aggressive treatment that the nurse views as merely prolonging the death process and creating unnecessary suffering
- Insufficient informed consent, such as might occur if the child's parents and other family members were not in agreement regarding the treatment plan
- Working with healthcare professionals that the nurse views as being incompetent

- Lack of consensus from either the healthcare team or the child's family on the treatment plan
- Lack of continuity of care in fulfilling the treatment plan
- Inappropriate use of resources, whether in terms of material supplies or manpower
- Providing care that the nurse views as not being in the best interest of the patient
- Failing to provide adequate pain relief
- Providing false hope to patients and their families
- Providing care that the nurse views as accelerating the death process
- Disregarding the wishes of the patient; this can occur when the treatment team does not recognize that the child can adequately express preferences

How can moral distress be managed in the workplace? Dos Santos et al. (2018) suggest that the emotional state of resilience can be particularly effective in resolving moral distress. **Resilience** is considered to be the ability of a person to respond to stress in a healthy way so that the worker is still able to achieve personal goals while experiencing little psychological or physical damage. Nurses can be encouraged to develop resilience through the use of strategies such as taking a few moments to reflect before talking with a child's family about a difficult healthcare situation, encouraging colleagues to emotionally support one another when caring for severely ill children, and promoting self-care of healthcare professionals through the development of interests outside of work to achieve a sense of balance.

What can organizations do to help pediatric nurses and healthcare workers cope with moral distress and develop resilience? There are several strategies that have been suggested by Dos Santos et al. (2018):

- encourage discussion of ethical dilemmas by healthcare team members through debriefing sessions
- promote use of consultations with the facility ethics committee to support the staff members who are dealing with the ethical dilemma
- implement use of ethical rounds to discuss the ethical dilemma before there is an escalation among stakeholders
- encourage healthcare professionals to recognize that moral distress is a sign of humanity and of having well-developed moral values

- provide healthcare team members with a work environment that has a policy of openness in which there is not a fear of reprisals when voicing an opinion

MORAL COURAGE

Just as pediatric nurses are particularly vulnerable to moral distress, they can also experience **moral courage**. Dos Santos et al. (2018) define this as a person's ability to overcome fear and fight for the values that he or she views as being most significant. The healthcare professional who chooses to exercise moral courage may, however, consequently experience conflict with colleagues and supervisory personnel in the workplace.

The development of moral courage in the pediatric nurse requires a commitment to ethical principles despite the presence of risks such as a threatened professional reputation, workplace isolation, and possible retaliation from colleagues. How can the pediatric nurse who may be faced with ethical dilemmas on a daily basis develop the moral courage needed to face them? Muehlbauer (2014) recommends that a nurse who is faced with confronting a moral dilemma develop a plan to address the situation. The plan can consist of agenda items such as realistically considering the consequences, discussing the situation with a trustworthy person who can be impartial and can provide a new perspective, and using calming exercises such as controlled deep breathing and visual imagery.

Moral courage develops each time the nurse takes a risk to overcome fear and fight for the values that are most important to him or her. An important part of moral courage is making the effort to express oneself assertively yet appropriately. Muehlbauer (2014) indicates that such an assertive message in the face of moral distress should consist of the following:

- a nonjudgmental explanation of the behavior change that the nurse is seeking
- a clear admission of the nurse's feelings in the situation
- an explanation of the effect of the other person's behavior that is leading to the nurse's moral distress
- a clear statement of behavior change that is being sought by the nurse

Ultimately, moral courage will develop through the use of negotiation skills. Each time the nurse confronts his or her fear and expresses moral distress in an assertive manner, the nurse develops additional resilience and consequent moral courage. As each morally distressing situation moves toward a more effective conclusion that will achieve positive patient care outcomes, the improved outcome serves as confirmation of the nurse's improved level of moral courage.

In summary, the chapter has reviewed some of the most common ethical issues that may be experienced by nurses who are caring for children or adolescent patients. As society changes, technology expands, and social media continues to explode, there will be new ethical challenges that will present themselves to healthcare providers and team members in years to come. Now that the foundation has been laid with a discussion of ethical issues that might occur with society's youngest patients, the following chapter will discuss ethical issues related to the oldest patients.

REFERENCES

Butts, J., & Rich, K. (2020). *Nursing ethics: Across the curriculum and into practice*. Jones and Bartlett Learning.

Carnevale, F. (2012). Ethical considerations in pediatric nursing. *Journal of the Brazilian Pediatric Nurses Society, 12*(1), 37–47.

Choe, K., Kim, Y., & Yang, Y. (2017). Pediatric nurses' ethical difficulties in the bedside care of children. *Nursing Ethics, 26*(2), 541–552. https://doi.org/10.1177/0969733017708330

Davis, M., & Fang, A. (2023). Emancipated minor. In *StatPearls* [Internet]. StatPearls Publishing. https://www.ncbi.nlm.nih.gov/books/NBK554594/

De Jesus, V., Liem, A., Borra, D., & Appel, J. (2022). Who's the boss? Ethical dilemmas in the treatment of children and adolescents. *Focus, 20*(2), 215–219. https://doi.org/10.1176/appi.focus.20210037

Dos Santos, R. P., Garros, D., & Carnevale, F. (2018). Difficult decisions in pediatric practice and moral distress in the intensive care unit. *Revista Brasileira de Terapia Intensiva, 30*(2), 226–232. https://doi.org/10.5935/0103-507X.20180039

Furingsten, L., Sjögren, R., & Forsner, M. (2015). Ethical challenges when caring for dying children. *Nursing Ethics, 22*(2), 176–187. https://doi.org/10.1177/0969733014533234

Muehlbauer, P. (2014, March 1). Have the moral courage to do the right thing. *ONSVoice*. https://www.ons.org/03-2014/have-moral-courage-do-right-thing

Ulrich, C. (2012). *Nursing ethics in everyday practice*. Sigma Theta Tau International.

NCLEX FORMAT REVIEW QUESTIONS

Match the items correctly.

a. potential cause of moral distress

b. strategy that may relieve moral distress

1. _____ working with healthcare professionals viewed by the nurse as being incompetent
2. _____ lack of continuity of care in implementing the treatment plan
3. _____ implementing ethical rounds to discuss the ethical dilemma before things escalate
4. _____ inappropriate use of resources, whether material supplies or manpower
5. _____ providing aggressive treatment that may prolong the dying process
6. _____ using consultations with the facility ethics committee to support staff members
7. _____ using debriefing sessions to encourage discussion of ethical dilemmas
8. _____ providing care that the nurse views as not being in the patient's best interest
9. _____ lack of consensus from the healthcare team or family on treatment plan
10. _____ providing the healthcare team with a work environment that has a policy of openness

Correct answers:

1. a	4. a	7. b	10. b
2. a	5. a	8. a	
3. b	6. b	9. a	

11. Select all of the individuals who would be considered to have emancipated minor status.
    a. _____ Sue, who is 17 years old and newly married
    b. _____ Bill, who is a month short of his 18th birthday and is active-duty military
    c. _____ John, who is a 16-year-old singer who manages his own finances
    d. _____ Angie, a 16-year-old single mother who is engaged to be married

Correct answer: a, b, c

12. The ability of the nurse to respond to stress so that the nurse can achieve personal goals while experiencing little psychological or physical damage from the stress is known as:

    a. ____ moral courage

    b. ____ ethical numbness

    c. ____ resilience

    d. ____ moral distress

Correct answer: c

13. A nurse is practicing under highly stressful conditions and is experiencing a heavy workload with the need to complete multiple tasks in a short period of time. The nurse is failing to follow approved protocol in order to complete as many tasks as possible. The nurse is most likely to be experiencing:

    a. ____ moral courage

    b. ____ ethical numbness

    c. ____ resilience

    d. ____ moral distress

Correct answer: b

14. A nurse is experiencing circumstances that are preventing him from doing what he knows to be the right thing to do in a specific situation. He is most likely experiencing:

    a. ____ moral courage

    b. ____ ethical numbness

    c. ____ resilience

    d. ____ moral distress

Correct answer: d

15. A nurse is able to overcome her fear and fight for the values that she views as being most significant. She is most likely experiencing:

    a. ____ moral courage

    b. ____ ethical numbness

    c. ____ resilience

    d. ____ moral distress

Correct answer: a

TEAM-BUILDING EXERCISE

Instructions: Divide students into teams of at least three people and preferably no more than five. Each person should have a role assigned in the exercise. One person will be the leader, one person will be the timekeeper, and one person will be the recorder. The **leader** will oversee helping the discussion progress so that the objectives of the exercise are accomplished. The **timekeeper** should intervene when necessary to keep the discussion focused on the topic of the exercise and should periodically remind team members of the amount of time remaining to complete the exercise. The **recorder** will be responsible for taking notes during the discussion that can be utilized when the exercise results are presented to the class. If additional team members are included in the group, one person can be assigned to assist with the note-taking and transcription process, and the additional person can assist the team leader in guiding the discussion and assist in preparing the final presentation of the results.

SCENARIO FOR TEAM-BUILDING EXERCISE

The Clarks are a married couple with three grown children. Two children are married with families of their own. One 17-year-old son, Jim, is mildly intellectually challenged and lives with Mr. and Mrs. Clark while also attending a day program to learn skills to help him ultimately live on his own. Jim was diagnosed with leukemia four years ago. He has undergone multiple cycles of chemotherapy. His primary provider recently told him and his parents that there is evidence that the cancer has spread. Jim has expressed to his nurse that he is tired of undergoing the treatments and would like to die peacefully. He mentions that his parents are completely against this and are trying to convince his physician that Jim is not able to make an informed decision.

QUESTIONS

1. Analyze the situation and discuss how Jim will be impacted by assent to treatment vs. informed consent.

2. Analyze the situation and discuss how Jim will be impacted by the three essential elements of informed consent.

3. Analyze the situation and discuss how Jim will be affected by the limits of confidentiality.

4. Analyze the situation and discuss the elements of Jim's situation that could cause his nurse to experience ethical numbness.

5. Analyze the situation and discuss the elements of Jim's situation that could cause his nurse to experience moral distress.

6. Analyze Jim's situation as well as that of his family. What could his nurse do to develop resilience?

7. Analyze Jim's situation as well as that of his family. What could his nurse do to develop moral courage?

CHAPTER 6

ETHICAL ISSUES PERTAINING TO OLDER ADULTS

CHAPTER OBJECTIVES

After studying this chapter, students will be able to:

- Discuss the importance of recognizing the older adult patient's right to autonomy as the nurse contributes to the treatment plan.
- Describe the ethical dilemma that may develop as the nurse observes the principle of beneficence in care of the older adult.
- Discuss the three sections of the process of obtaining an informed consent from the older adult patient.
- Describe principlism as an ethical framework in care of older adults.
- Discuss how the nurse can protect the older adult patient's right to self-determination.
- Discuss moral agency as it applies to care of the older adult.
- Compare and contrast decisional capacity with paternalism as they relate to care of the older adult.
- Discuss characteristics of an individual who has been shown to be incompetent to make decisions.
- Analyze the importance of the doctrine of double effect in developing a treatment plan for an older adult patient.
- Analyze the relationship of compassion and ethical sensitivity and their importance as the nurse provides care to the older adult.

KEY TERMS

autonomy
beneficence
compassion
competence

decisional capacity
doctrine of double effect
ethical sensitivity
informed consent
moral agency
nonmaleficence
paternalism
principlism
right to self-determination
threshold
voluntariness

The longevity of older adults is increasing at an unprecedented level across the globe as medicine becomes more capable of managing the intricacies of multiple chronic conditions in a patient. However, just as medical challenges must be managed to provide the most effective care for this population of patients, ethical challenges must also be overcome. For example, maintaining the patient's **autonomy** is essential, since the patient has a right to make decisions about his or her own care through informed consent. This can be difficult when an older adult has a cognitive impairment. Consequently, the healthcare team must balance the patient's right to autonomy with the need to protect the person from harm due to their diminished capability to make appropriate decisions. In comparison, the principle of **beneficence**, which obligates the healthcare team to act in the patient's best interest, may inadvertently create an ethical dilemma as nurses struggle to balance aggressive medical treatments with the expressed wishes of the patient and family members. Additional risk to the patient may develop in violation of the principle of **nonmaleficence**, which requires nurses to literally "do no harm." As healthcare providers increasingly treat older adults' chronic conditions with multiple medications, nurses may struggle to balance the need to achieve the highest possible patient care outcomes with the polypharmacy that may be occurring (Alodhialah et al., 2024).

INFORMED CONSENT

As previously mentioned, maintaining the older adult's right to autonomy is vital, particularly as the patient must be able to make informed decisions regarding consent for treatment. This can be challenging if the patient is experiencing signs and/or symptoms of cognitive impairment. Crane et al. (2004) has indicated that there are three distinct sections to the process of obtaining an **informed consent**.

Threshold—these are the preconditions that exist prior to obtaining the informed consent. Both **competence** and **voluntariness** are included in this area. Competence includes the ability to make a decision as well as the ability to gather new information and relate it to the person's individual values and goals. Voluntariness cannot exist when there is any evidence of coercion, persuasion, or manipulation on the part of either the healthcare team members or the patient's support system.

Information—this stage consists of both disclosure of information and understanding of the information presented. The language of the consent form can be crucial at this point. If the form is worded at too high a reading level, the patient may not be able to comprehend it. In both the threshold and the information stages, sufficient time should be provided to ensure that the older adult who is experiencing age-related changes such as a decrease in short-term memory can adequately process the information. Be aware that the more detailed the informed consent form becomes, the more anxiety and confusion may be produced in the older adult who is struggling to comprehend it due to cognitive changes. If the consent form must be extensive and detailed, consider dividing the form into sections and discuss one section per session. Determine the presence of age-related vision and hearing changes that can influence the patient's seeming failure to comprehend information. If visual acuity is diminished, consider enlarging the form's print, changing the font, or even reading the form aloud to the patient. Prior to initiating the informed consent process, make certain to assess the presence of diminished hearing so that hearing aids from the patient's home setting can be obtained or even a lower voice tone used when reading the form aloud.

Consent—this stage includes the formal decision-making process related to participation in treatment. Assess the patient's support network to determine whether family participation in the consent process will facilitate the older adult patient's completion of the form.

TABLE 6.1 STAGES OF THE INFORMED CONSENT PROCESS

Stage of Informed Consent	Description
threshold	These are preconditions existing prior to obtaining informed consent. Both competence and voluntariness are included. Competence encompasses the ability to decide and ability to gather new information and relate it to values and goals. Voluntariness cannot exist when there is evidence of coercion, persuasion, or manipulation.

(Continued)

TABLE 6.1 *(Continued)*

Stage of Informed Consent	Description
information	This stage consists of both disclosure and understanding of information. Language of the consent form can be crucial. Sufficient time should be provided to ensure that an older adult experiencing decreased short-term memory can process the information. If the consent form is extensive and detailed, consider dividing the form into sections and discuss one section per session. Determine the presence of age-related vision and hearing changes.
consent	This stage is the formal decision-making process. Assess the patient's support network to determine whether family participation in the consent process will facilitate the older adult patient's completion of the form.

ETHICAL FRAMEWORK

Intrinsic to the process of obtaining informed consent is the determination of the older adult patient's decision-making capacity. This will involve maintaining a balance between respect for the patient's autonomy and the need to protect a person who may not have sufficient capacity to refrain from making harmful decisions. The most common ethical framework used in healthcare decisions involving older adults is **principlism**, which uses as its guiding principles autonomy, nonmaleficence, beneficence, and justice. Autonomy can be encouraged through the use of advance healthcare directives so that the patient's wishes are known even if the person becomes incapacitated. The preferences of the older adult patient, including those who are experiencing cognitive impairment, should be respected unless illness is clearly impairing decision-making capacity. These preferences include the patient's right to refuse treatment, even if that treatment could prolong life. Obtaining a valid informed consent helps protect the older adult's **right to self-determination** since it requires a competent person to make a choice of his or her own volition without being influenced and after receiving adequate information. The patient's self-determination can be increased through the use of shared decision-making in which the patient and the members of the healthcare team work together to make decisions affecting the patient. (Kotzé, 2022).

While the members of the healthcare team should respect the older adult patient's right to autonomy, they must also be cognizant of the need to provide care that benefits the patients while also preventing harm from occurring. In an effort to give priority to the principles of beneficence and nonmaleficence, nurses must ensure that patients are aware that they can refuse any treatment considered as part of the plan and should consequently be made aware of potential side effects, risks, and also possible benefits. Verify that explanations consider the patient's knowledge level and reading level, and schedule follow-up sessions as needed. This may be particularly important when the patient and family or support system must make decisions regarding withdrawal of treatment (Kotzé, 2022).

Part of the healthcare team's respect for the older adult's right to autonomy is the respect for the patient's right to make deliberate choices. This is based on the individual's **moral agency**, which refers to the recognition that each person has the responsibility for directing his or her own beliefs and actions. Moral agency is related to **decisional capacity**, which is each person's ability to come to reasonable conclusions and is often considered along with competence. In contrast to this is **paternalism**, which occurs when a member of the healthcare team makes choices for a patient based on what the health professional believes would be best for the patient rather than based on the expressed needs and desires of the patient. Nurses must be cognizant of the fact that the older adult patient is particularly vulnerable to experiencing paternalism because of the erroneous view that older adults are not capable of making decisions for themselves (Butts & Rich, 2020). According to Beauchamp and Childress (2013), the incompetent individual frequently exhibits:

- inability to communicate preferences
- inability to understand the consequences of the present situation
- inability to understand information that is particularly relevant
- inability to provide reasons that are rational, reasonable, and related to either risks or benefits

The **doctrine of double effect** is vital when making decisions regarding a treatment plan for older adults that is ethically appropriate. This principle indicates that an action is permissible if a good effect is intended, the bad effect is foreseen but not intended, and other preexisting conditions are met (Brueck & Sulmasy, 2020). This is especially necessary when the older adult patient is experiencing potentially debilitating symptoms such as extreme pain. The healthcare team's goal will be to mitigate the pain as much as possible without leading to a loss of function for the patient or potentially hastening death.

In order for the healthcare team members to provide care that respects all ethical principles, the concepts of **compassion** and **ethical sensitivity** must be implemented into the care provision. Blomqvist et al. (2023) notes that *compassion* literally means a deep awareness of another person's suffering that leads to a motivation to help the person. In comparison, ethical sensitivity is the caregiver's ability to recognize the ethical aspects of a situation and is the prerequisite for reflection, decision-making, and ultimately action. Ethical sensitivity in the caregiver involves being able to recognize patient alterations, exhibit compassion in response to the patient's needs, show respect for the patient, and respect the patient's right to self-determination. Ethical sensitivity requires the caregiver to be responsive to the needs of the patient while also recognizing what the patient considers to be most meaningful. It is preceded by compassion for the patient, and it is compassion that forms the basis for the interaction between the patient and the nurse. Ethical sensitivity allows the older adult to feel that they are being heard and are being allowed to make their own decisions regarding their care and treatment plan. The caregiver offers a person-centered approach, and it is ethical sensitivity that makes this possible (Blomqvist et al., 2023).

In summary, the nurse who is providing care for older adult patients must be able to balance the compassion and ethical sensitivity needed when caring for this particularly vulnerable group of individuals with recognition of the need to respect the older adult patient's need for autonomy and self-determination. This ability will also be needed when caring for patients who are nearing the end of their lives and will be discussed in the subsequent chapter.

REFERENCES

Alodhialah, A. M., Almutairi, A. A., & Almutairi, M. (2024). Ethical and legal challenges in caring for older adults with multimorbidities: Best practices for nurses. *Healthcare, 12*(16), 1585. https://doi.org/10.3390/healthcare12161585

Beauchamp, T. L., & Childress, J. F. (2013). *Principles of biomedical ethics.* (7th ed.). Oxford University Press.

Blomqvist, H., Bergdahl, E., & Hemberg, J. (2023). Ethical sensitivity and compassion in home care: Leaders' views. *Nursing Ethics, 30*(2), 180–196. https://doi.org/10.1177/09697330221122965

Brueck, M., & Sulmasy, D. (2020). The rule of double effect. *Health Policy and Law.* https://bioethics.hms.harvard.edu/journal/rule-double-effect

Butts, J., & Rich, K. (2020). *Nursing ethics: Across the curriculum and into practice.* Jones and Bartlett Learning.

Crane, P. B., Cody, M., & McSweeney, J. (2004). Informed consent: A process to facilitate older adults' participation in research. *Journal of Gerontological Nursing, 30*(4), 40–44. https://doi.org/10.3928/0098-9134-20040401-09

Kotzé, C., & Roos, J. L. (2022). Ageism, human rights and ethical aspects of end-of-life care for older people with serious mental illness. *Front Psychiatry, 13*, 906873. https://doi.org/10.3389/fpsyt.2022.906873

NCLEX FORMAT REVIEW QUESTIONS

1. Principlism includes: (Select all that apply)

   a. ____ fidelity
   b. ____ autonomy
   c. ____ veracity
   d. ____ nonmaleficence
   e. ____ paternalism
   f. ____ beneficence
   g. ____ equality
   h. ____ justice

   Correct answer: b, d, f, h

2. A member of the healthcare team makes a choice for the patient based on what the health professional believes would be best for the patient rather than on the patient's verbalized needs. This is known as:

   a. ____ moral agency
   b. ____ principlism
   c. ____ paternalism
   d. ____ decisional capacity

   Correct answer: c

Match the section of the process of obtaining an informed consent with the correct description.

a. consent
b. information
c. threshold

1. ____ consists of both disclosure and understanding of information
2. ____ includes the formal decision-making process
3. ____ assess the patient for vision and hearing changes
4. ____ includes both competence and voluntariness
5. ____ language of the form is most crucial at this point

6. _____ assess the patient's support network to facilitate form completion
7. _____ consists of the preconditions that exist before obtaining consent
8. _____ assess for evidence of coercion, persuasion, or manipulation

Correct answers:

1. b	3. b	5. b	7. c
2. a	4. c	6. a	8. c

TEAM-BUILDING EXERCISE

Instructions: Divide students into teams of at least three people and preferably no more than five. Each person should have a role assigned in the exercise. One person will be the leader, one person will be the timekeeper, and one person will be the recorder. The **leader** will oversee helping the discussion progress so that the objectives of the exercise are accomplished. The **timekeeper** should intervene when necessary to keep the discussion focused on the topic of the exercise and should periodically remind team members of the amount of time remaining to complete the exercise. The **recorder** will be responsible for taking notes during the discussion that can be utilized when the exercise results are presented to the class. If additional team members are included in the group, one person can be assigned to assist with the note-taking and transcription process, and the additional person can assist the team leader in guiding the discussion and assist in preparing the final presentation of the results.

SCENARIO FOR TEAM-BUILDING EXERCISE

Mrs. Pearson is an 84-year-old female who has been experiencing occasional episodes of chest pain. She does not show any evidence of mental decline but does have bilateral hearing deficits that have been corrected with hearing aids. She also has cataracts, which are scheduled to be removed in a month. She speaks English as a second language, having immigrated to the United States as a child. Mrs. Pearson notified her primary healthcare provider of the episodes of chest pain, and she was referred to a cardiologist. The cardiologist wants to perform a cardiac catheterization on her this week. Mrs. Pearson was stunned by the urgency with which the procedure was scheduled and called her daughter to discuss the situation. The daughter informed Mrs. Pearson that she will be arriving in her city during the upcoming weekend to further discuss things and told her "not to sign anything until I read it first."

QUESTIONS

1. Analyze Mrs. Pearson's situation and discuss how her right to autonomy can be maintained.

2. Analyze Mrs. Pearson's situation and determine how the threshold section of the informed consent process applies to her.

3. Analyze Mrs. Pearson's situation and determine how the information section of the informed consent process applies to her.

4. Analyze Mrs. Pearson's situation and determine what could be done by the nurse to expedite signing of the informed consent for cardiac catheterization.

5. Analyze Mrs. Pearson's situation and determine how the ethical framework of principlism applies to her.

6. Analyze Mrs. Pearson's situation and determine what the nurse could do to adhere to the patient's right to self-determination.

7. Analyze Mrs. Pearson's situation and discuss how she would be affected by moral agency and decisional capacity.

8. Analyze Mrs. Pearson's situation and discuss examples of paternalism that are noted. How could each one be resolved in a way that provides the most benefit to the patient?

9. Analyze Mrs. Pearson's situation and discuss how she would be impacted by the doctrine of double effect.

10. What could the healthcare team do to demonstrate the maximum amount of ethical sensitivity in Mrs. Pearson's care?

CHAPTER 7

ETHICAL ISSUES PERTAINING TO END-OF-LIFE CARE

CHAPTER OBJECTIVES

After studying this chapter, students will be able to:

- Explain the various aspects of the Patient Self-Determination Act.
- Compare and contrast the various forms of advance directives and explain their relevance to end-of-life care in a patient.
- Discuss healthcare power of attorney and the relationship to a patient experiencing end-of-life care.
- Explain the responsibilities of a healthcare surrogate.
- Compare and contrast a living will with a do-not-resuscitate order.
- Discuss the ethical principle of beneficence and explain its relevance to end-of-life care.
- Discuss the ethical principle of justice and explain its relevance to the patient receiving end-of-life care.
- Discuss the ethical principle of fidelity and explain its relevance to the patient receiving end-of-life care.
- Discuss the concept of medical futility and explain its relevance to the patient receiving end-of-life care.
- Discuss the process a healthcare provider should follow when challenged by the need to withdraw treatment from a patient receiving end-of-life care.

KEY TERMS

autonomy
beneficence
do-not-resuscitate order
fidelity
healthcare power of attorney
healthcare proxy

justice
living will
medical futility
Patient Self-Determination Act
Physician Orders for Life-Sustaining Treatment

The provision of end-of-life care can be fraught with ethical land mines for the nurse who is unfamiliar with the nuances of ethical principles and the legislation that energized legal decisions regarding those principles. A major ethical principle that forms the foundation for end-of-life care is that of **autonomy**. As noted in previous chapters, autonomy is essentially the freedom as well as the ability to act in a self-determined manner (Butts & Rich, 2020). The principle is the cornerstone of the **Patient Self-Determination Act**, legislation proposed in 1990, that mandates that healthcare facilities inform patients of their right to be involved in making decisions about the medical care that they receive. The legislation also required patients to be asked about advance directives by healthcare staff members, who are required to document each patient's wishes regarding care (Teoli & Ghassemzadeh, 2023). Ethical dilemmas can develop for healthcare team members who struggle to implement the patient's wishes regarding end-of-life care when, as healthcare providers, they have taken an oath to uphold and sustain human life.

ADVANCE DIRECTIVES

Advance directives are legal documents that describe a patient's preferences regarding medical decisions. The documents indicate the healthcare options that the person accepts or rejects, both in the present and in future circumstances. Individuals are also designated who will serve as spokespersons on the patient's behalf if the patient can't communicate his or her preferences. Forms of advance directives can include:

- Physician Orders for Life-Sustaining Treatment (POLST)
- Medical Orders for Life-Sustaining Treatment (MOLST)
- Medical Orders for Scope of Treatment (MOST)
- Physician Orders for Scope of Treatment (POST)
- Do-Not-Resuscitate Order (DNR)
- Clinician Orders for Life-Sustaining Treatment (COLST)
- Transportable Physician Orders for Patient Preferences (TPOPP)

These can vary from state to state (House et al., 2023).

HEALTHCARE POWER OF ATTORNEY

As mentioned in a previous chapter, a **healthcare power of attorney** or **healthcare proxy** is a healthcare surrogate who is authorized to make medical decisions on behalf of a patient who is unable to indicate his or her wishes and thus functions as an advance directive. The surrogate is expected to make decisions based on knowledge of what the patient would want done in similar circumstances. Although typically a legal guardian, spouse, adult child, or parent is able to act as a surrogate, some states allow any person who has a close relationship with the patient to serve in this capacity. The patient will maintain his or her autonomy to make healthcare-related decisions as long as he or she shows competency and the ability to make decisions. Once the patient can no longer communicate his or her wishes, the healthcare provider must begin collaborating with the healthcare surrogate. If no surrogate has been designated, the provider must act in the best interest of the patient using professional judgment. If an ethical dilemma arises, the healthcare facility's ethics committee can be utilized to provide guidance in resolving the issue (House et al., 2023).

LIVING WILL

A **living will** can be completed by an individual to indicate healthcare preferences. This advance directive document usually discusses the person's choice regarding cardiopulmonary resuscitation (CPR) and mechanical ventilation. In addition, it may address the use of feeding tubes and blood products, as well as other options. As part of the patient's right to self-determination, he or she can refuse any form of treatment, even those treatments that may prolong life. In order for a living will to be implemented, there usually is a requirement for one or more physicians to indicate that the patient is experiencing an illness that has a terminal prognosis. However, the specific requirements for implementation of living wills can vary from state to state (House et al., 2023).

PHYSICIAN ORDERS

A **do-not-resuscitate order** is a document signed by the patient's healthcare provider that expresses the patient's desire to avoid efforts to resuscitate him or her should his or her condition sufficiently deteriorate. The patient can specify which resuscitative measures he or she will be willing to accept. In comparison, the **Physician Orders for Life-Sustaining Treatment** form can actually contradict a preexisting living will and in some states can replace the living will since it is more flexible and can be adjusted more easily in response to changes in the patient's condition. In addition, a surrogate can complete the Physician Orders for Life-Sustaining Treatment form rather than the patient. Whether the patient chooses a do-not-resuscitate order or comfort measures only, the person can still receive comfort care, pain management, and measures to minimize suffering. As the nurse and the members of the healthcare team implement the patient's advance directives, an ethical dilemma can result. The nurse may struggle with withholding lifesaving measures such as feeding tubes and blood products because of the patient's expressed wishes in a living will (House et al., 2023).

Table 7.1 shows a comparison between the various types of advance directives.

TABLE 7.1 COMPARISON OF ADVANCE DIRECTIVES

Advance Directive	Description
healthcare power of attorney	Healthcare surrogate who is authorized to make medical decisions on behalf of a patient who is unable to indicate his or her wishes; typically, a legal guardian, spouse, adult child, or parent
living will	Completed by a person to indicate healthcare preferences; document usually discusses the person's choice regarding CPR, mechanical ventilation, feeding tubes, and blood products
do-not-resuscitate order	Document signed by the healthcare provider that expresses the patient's desire to avoid efforts to resuscitate him or her if condition deteriorates sufficiently; the patient can specify which resuscitative measures can be utilized
Physician Orders for Life-Sustaining Treatment	Form can contradict a preexisting living will and can be completed by a surrogate; whether the patient chooses a do-not-resuscitate order or comfort measures only, the person can still receive comfort care, pain management, and measures to minimize suffering.

BENEFICENCE

In addition to autonomy, **beneficence** is another ethical principle that ensures that nurses defend implementation of the most useful intervention for the patient. Healthcare providers may not always be aware of the patient's wishes regarding end-of-life care. If the patient is not able to participate in the decision-making process or hasn't documented his or her wishes for end-of-life care, decisions will be made by the provider in consultation with the patient, relatives, or the patient's healthcare proxy. The responsibility of the nurse and the healthcare team will be to advocate for the treatment plan that will provide the patient with the highest quality of care possible throughout the dying process (Akdeniz et al., 2021).

JUSTICE

In comparison to beneficence is the ethical principle of **justice**, which states that team members have an obligation to ethically promote appropriate treatment for patients approaching the end of life. If the patient requires resources that have limited availability, are difficult to locate, or must be administered by a select number of highly trained personnel, healthcare providers may experience an ethical dilemma as they struggle to provide equal access to all patients requiring the resources (Akdeniz et al., 2021).

FIDELITY

Another ethical dilemma may develop as healthcare team members struggle with implementing the ethical principle of **fidelity**, which requires providers to be honest with patients undergoing end-of-life care about their disease processes. Fidelity is a close relative of autonomy since that principle cannot be respected without the patient receiving the truth about the disease and its likely outcome. Team members may struggle with the obligation to provide the patient with full knowledge of the disease process and likely consequences of treatment options if family members are providing opposition to this. Also, occasionally the patient may not want complete details about his or her prognosis as the disease process progresses. Such a request should be handled with tact and sensitivity so that the provider can be ready to provide additional information to the patient at any point when the patient is ready to receive it (Akdeniz et al., 2021).

MEDICAL FUTILITY

Hospice and palliative care nurses have identified **medical futility** as an ethical issue when caring for patients at the end of their lives. Futile treatments can lead to the patient experiencing increased pain, loss of dignity, and decreased quality of life, as well as increasing anxiety for members of the patient's support system (Cheon et al., 2015). Just as the nurse can experience an ethical dilemma when asked to withhold nutrition from a dying patient who has requested this as part of an advance directive, another dilemma can develop if the patient insists on receiving a treatment that won't be beneficial. In this case, the healthcare provider should tactfully explain why the treatment would not be effective but might in fact result in further pain and suffering for the patient (Akdeniz et al., 2021).

WITHDRAWING TREATMENT

The healthcare provider's decision to withdraw life-sustaining interventions can create an ethical dilemma for the nurse as he or she struggles to carry out the order. While the patient who has decision-making capacity can ask at any time that any medical intervention be stopped, the patient who lacks appropriate capacity will require a surrogate to assist in decision-making. The healthcare provider should determine the patient's goals of care and preferences regarding life-sustaining interventions as early in the treatment plan as possible so that the patient has full decisional capacity for the extent of the disease process. When challenged by a decision regarding the need to withdraw life-sustaining treatment from a patient receiving end-of-life care, the healthcare provider should do the following:

- Review with the patient his or her advance directive, if one exists. If there is no advance directive, discuss the patient's values as well as both goals and preferences for treatment. If the patient has designated a surrogate to assist in the decision-making process, include that person in the discussion.
- Document what the patient has expressed regarding preferences and also identify the patient's surrogate if one has been designated. If the patient has completed an advance directive or a durable power of attorney for healthcare, make certain that a copy of these documents is included.
- Provide all relevant medical information to the patient, as well as the surrogate if applicable, to support the decision-making process.
- Review with the patient and surrogate if applicable the possibility of initiating an intervention and evaluating its clinical effectiveness after a specified period of time to determine whether there has been improvement. Emphasize that if the intervention has not

achieved the goals that were agreed upon, it can be withdrawn at any point.

- Make certain that the patient and the surrogate if applicable are reassured that all medically appropriate care will be provided. If the patient has requested symptom management and aggressive palliative care, that will be provided as well.
- If a surrogate is relevant, explain both to that person and to the patient that the surrogate will make decisions to withhold or withdraw life-sustaining interventions if the patient lacks decision-making capacity.
- Consult with an ethics committee when:
  - The patient or applicable surrogate cannot reach agreement with the healthcare team about a decision to withdraw life-sustaining treatment,
  - The patient no longer has decision-making capacity and there is no longer a surrogate available to act on the patient's behalf, or
  - The patient's healthcare provider judges that a decision by the patient's surrogate is in violation of the patient's values, goals, and preferences for treatment or is not in the patient's best interest medically.
- Ensure that relevant standards for clinical practice and palliative care are followed by the healthcare team when implementing a decision to withdraw any intervention that could potentially sustain life (American Medical Association, n.d.).

In summary, all nurses should be familiar with the various forms of advance directives that exist in his or her states of licensure. The increased knowledge regarding these may help in avoiding an ethical dilemma that makes caring for a terminally ill patient all the more difficult. Some of the information discussed in this chapter pertaining to patient capacity to determine wishes and the use of a healthcare surrogate will be helpful as we move into the subsequent chapter regarding ethical issues pertaining to the care of psychiatric patients.

REFERENCES

Akdeniz, M., Yardımcı, B., & Kavukcu, E. (2021). Ethical considerations at the end-of-life care. *SAGE Open Medicine, 9*. https://doi.org/10.1177/20503121211000918

American Medical Association. (n.d.). Medical ethics. Retrieved May 3, 2025, from https://code-medical-ethics.ama-assn.org/

Butts, J., & Rich, K. (2020). *Nursing ethics: Across the curriculum and into practice.* Jones and Bartlett Learning.

Cheon, J., Coyle, N., Wiegand, D., & Welsh, S. (2015). Ethical issues experienced by hospice and palliative nurses. *Journal of Hospice & Palliative Nursing, 17*(1), 7–13. https://doi.org/10.1097/NJH.0000000000000129

House, S. A., Schoo, C., & Ogilvie, W. A. (2023). Advance directives. In *StatPearls* [Internet]. StatPearls Publishing. https://www.ncbi.nlm.nih.gov/books/NBK459133/

Teoli, D., & Ghassemzadeh, S. (2023). Patient Self-Determination Act. In *StatPearls* [Internet]. StatPearls Publishing. https://www.ncbi.nlm.nih.gov/books/NBK538297/

NCLEX FORMAT REVIEW QUESTIONS

1. The freedom as well as the ability to act in a self-determined manner is a description of the ethical principle of:

    a. beneficence

    b. autonomy

    c. justice

    d. fidelity

Correct answer: b

2. The ethical principle that requires that medical resources be distributed fairly and that healthcare providers be impartial in delivering health services is known as:

    a. beneficence

    b. autonomy

    c. justice

    d. fidelity

Correct answer: c

3. The ethical principle that ensures nurses defend the implementation of the most useful intervention for the patient is known as:

    a. beneficence

    b. autonomy

    c. justice

    d. fidelity

Correct answer: a

4. The obligation of healthcare team members to be honest with patients undergoing end-of-life care about their disease processes is a description of the ethical principle known as:

   a. beneficence

   b. autonomy

   c. justice

   d. fidelity

   Correct answer: d

Match the advance directive with its correct description from the choices below.

5. _____ healthcare proxy
6. _____ living will
7. _____ Physician Orders for Life-Sustaining Treatment
8. _____ do-not-resuscitate order

   a. Healthcare provider tactfully explains why the treatment would not be effective but might in fact result in further pain and suffering for the patient

   b. Document signed by the healthcare provider that expresses the patient's desire to avoid efforts to resuscitate him or her if condition deteriorates sufficiently; the patient can specify which resuscitative measures can be utilized

   c. Document completed by a person to indicate healthcare preferences; the document usually discusses the person's choices regarding CPR, mechanical ventilation, feeding tubes, and blood products

   d. Healthcare surrogate who is authorized to make medical decisions on behalf of a patient who is unable to indicate his or her wishes, typically a legal guardian, spouse, adult child, or parent

   e. Document that can contradict a preexisting living will and can be completed by a surrogate; whether the patient chooses a do-not-resuscitate order or comfort measures only, the person can still receive comfort care, pain management, and measures to minimize suffering

Correct answers:

5. d
6. c
7. e
8. b

TEAM-BUILDING EXERCISE

Instructions: Divide students into teams of at least three people and preferably no more than five. Each person should have a role assigned in the exercise. One person will be the leader, one person will be the timekeeper, and one person will be the recorder. The **leader** will oversee helping the discussion progress so that the objectives of the exercise are accomplished. The **timekeeper** should intervene when necessary to keep the discussion focused on the topic of the exercise and should periodically remind team members of the amount of time remaining to complete the exercise. The **recorder** will be responsible for taking notes during the discussion that can be utilized when the exercise results are presented to the class. If additional team members are included in the group, one person can be assigned to assist with the notetaking and transcription process, and the additional person can assist the team leader in guiding the discussion and assist in preparing the final presentation of the results.

SCENARIO FOR TEAM-BUILDING EXERCISE

Mr. Smith is a 60-year-old married adult male who is in the last stages of a neurodegenerative disease, although he remains completely alert and oriented. He began to show symptoms of the disease approximately 5 years ago, and the symptoms began to intensify 3 years ago. He became bedbound last month and is expected to be ventilator-dependent within days. He has a living will that indicates he does not want to be resuscitated. His only relative, other than a brother who lives out of state, is his wife. Mrs. Smith has healthcare power of attorney for her husband.

QUESTIONS

1. Mr. Smith is still able to speak a few words and has indicated that he does not want to be resuscitated in any way. He also refused his doctor's suggestion of a feeding tube. Discuss the ethical dilemma that may develop for the nurse caring for Mr. Smith.

2. The nurse finds Mrs. Smith weeping. Mrs. Smith says, "I just can't carry out what he wants! He wants the IVs stopped, but I can't let that happen! It will be just like I've killed him!" Discuss the ethical dilemma that may develop for the nurse caring for Mr. Smith.

3. Mr. Smith has asked the physician for withdrawal of all medical treatment. Explain the process that should be initiated based on the patient's request.

4. Mrs. Smith asks the healthcare provider about a radical new treatment for her husband's disease that she has heard about being used currently in Europe. It has had very little testing completed, and most patients who have utilized it have died. Discuss what the provider should say to Mrs. Smith about this radical treatment.

5. Mr. Smith's brother arrives from out of state. He decides that his brother is not receiving adequate care and tells the provider that he wants a Physician Orders for Life-Sustaining Treatment document to be written. Discuss what the provider should tell the brother regarding this situation.

6. Discuss how the nurse can most appropriately demonstrate the ethical principle of fidelity in the care delivered to Mr. Smith and his family members.

7. Discuss how the nurse can most appropriately demonstrate the ethical principle of justice in the care delivered to Mr. Smith and his family members.

8. Mr. Smith's brother has several arguments with Mrs. Smith regarding the patient's care. The brother indicates that he may have his attorney sue Mrs. Smith to prevent her from exercising healthcare power of attorney to control Mr. Smith's care. Discuss the ethical dilemma that may develop for the nurse caring for Mr. Smith during this time.

CHAPTER 8

ETHICAL ISSUES PERTAINING TO NURSING CARE OF PSYCHIATRIC PATIENTS

CHAPTER OBJECTIVES

After studying this chapter, students will be able to:

- Discuss the ethical principles involved in mental healthcare.
- Define decisional capacity
- Describe how the mental healthcare team will determine decisional capacity.
- Describe the difference between comparative reasoning and consequential reasoning.
- Compare shared decision-making to collaborative decision-making.
- Discuss the model of supportive decision-making.
- Analyze the ethical dilemmas that could result during nursing care of psychiatric patients.
- Compare a duty to warn with a duty to protect.
- Describe the Tarasoff principle.
- Discuss the conditions under which a clinician must implement a duty to protect.

KEY TERMS

autonomy
beneficence
capacity
collaborative decision-making
comparative reasoning
competence

consequential reasoning
duty to protect
duty to warn
fidelity
integrity
justice
nonmaleficence
shared decision-making
Tarasoff principle
veracity

THE SUICIDAL PATIENT

The nurse caring for patients who are experiencing mental illness is particularly subject to experiencing ethical challenges, particularly if patients must be restrained because of violent or aggressive outbursts or if there are questions regarding the person's capacity to make rational, evidence-based decisions for him- or herself regarding care. If the patient's behavior requires coercion to be utilized, an ethical challenge for the nurse will be to assess the balance between beneficence and maleficence (Hem et al., 2018).

The likelihood of an ethical dilemma developing is especially high when the patient is suicidal. According to the National Institute of Mental Health (n.d.), the Centers for Disease Control and Prevention reported that, as of 2022, suicide was ranked as the eleventh leading cause of death for the population in the United States, resulting in more than 49,400 deaths annually. There were almost twice as many suicides in America as homicides.

The nurse who is caring for a suicidal patient can easily experience an ethical dilemma because of the difficulty in estimating risk for suicide. If suicidal risk is overestimated, the patient may be deprived of the right to self-govern, whereas if the risk is underestimated, at best the patient's safety is jeopardized and may result in the patient's successful suicide attempt. The need to gauge to some degree the patient's risk for suicide can produce an ethical dilemma for the nurse because of the involvement of multiple ethical principles, all of which have been discussed in previous chapters:

- **Autonomy**—the ability to self-govern
- **Beneficence**—acting in a way that produces the greatest benefit to the patient
- **Fidelity**—faithfully promoting the best interest of the patient
- **Integrity**—acting in an honorable manner within the healthcare profession
- **Justice**—providing fair treatment without evidence of prejudice
- **Nonmaleficence**—avoiding harm to the patient
- **Veracity**—being truthful with the patient (Bernert & Roberts, 2012)

Respect for the ethical principles of autonomy, veracity, and beneficence can be shown with the patient at risk for suicide through utilization of informed consent. This consists of informing the patient of the process to be utilized in evaluating his or her risk level, the assessment procedure, and the process of managing the risk for suicide. It involves the patient as a collaborator in the treatment process while also establishing the ethical responsibilities of the healthcare team and the basic rules of the process of maintaining the safety of the patient. It demonstrates a respect for the rights of the individual and the overall autonomy of the person while also establishing clear-cut boundaries (Bernert & Roberts, 2012).

The therapeutic nurse-patient relationship can be strengthened as sufficient time and effort are dedicated to answering the patient's questions about, for example, the suicide risk assessment, how the information gathered will be used, and the measures taken to maintain confidentiality. The nurse should recognize that patients will be asked to disclose the presence of symptoms that will indicate the extent of the disease process and may be experiencing fear of being stigmatized and labeled. Educating the patient regarding information on symptoms, the accuracy of a diagnosis, and his or her role as a partner in the treatment plan can empower the patient while also demonstrating veracity and fidelity (Bernert & Roberts, 2012).

DECISIONAL CAPACITY

Part of the process of obtaining an informed consent from a patient in order to initiate treatment is the determination of **capacity**. This refers to a person's ability to make decisions about a specific choice. This is not synonymous with **competence**, which is a legal term pertaining to a person's right to make his or her own decisions. If the patient is lacking capacity, state law will determine who has legal authority to speak for the patient; this may have been previously determined in an advance directive such as a durable healthcare power of attorney. The determination of a healthcare provider can be vital in interactions with the patient's family if family members disagree with the patient's choice or request an intervention that is not consistent with the wishes of the patient. If the patient hasn't arranged advance planning, state law may require a surrogate decision-maker to be named, and a guardian may be appointed. The patient must be determined to be legally incompetent before a guardianship petition can be fulfilled. Dementia-related illnesses such as Alzheimer's disease as well as some psychiatric disorders can be associated with impaired capacity of the patient (Doyle & Sollins, 2023).

A formal process of determining the patient's capacity may be utilized, particularly if the healthcare provider believes that family members may be likely to question findings. A face-to-face interview with the patient will usually be conducted and will assess four areas:

- Understanding—can the patient understand the information related to the treatment plan and the overall diagnosis?
- Appreciation—is the patient able to relate the information about the treatment plan and diagnosis to his or her own situation, particularly in terms of the potential benefits and harm?
- Reasoning—can the patient rationally evaluate the treatment alternatives as well as the diagnosis in terms of the ratio of risk to potential benefits, particularly in consideration of the impact on activities of daily living?
- Choice—can the patient clearly communicate a decision about his or her willingness or reluctance to participate in recommended treatments or tests?

Documentation of the four areas regarding a specific choice, such as a treatment option, for example, is essential to the assessment of capacity. Also important is the presence of **comparative reasoning**, which is the ability to compare treatment options, as well as **consequential reasoning**, which is the ability to understand what it means to select an option from those offered (Doyle & Sollins, 2023).

SUPPORTED DECISION-MAKING

An approach to assisting the mental health patient who is exhibiting decreased decisional capacity is **shared decision-making**. This is a process of decision-making that occurs jointly between the healthcare team and the patient. The process will be based on a relationship having developed between the healthcare professional and the patient so that the team member will help the patient understand the various options that are available for proposed treatment along with advantages and disadvantages, make recommendations to the patient, and help the patient base his or her choice on the highest-quality evidence available. This model of decision-making involves both the healthcare team and the patient providing each other with all available information pertaining to the proposed treatment so that a mutually agreeable consensus can be reached regarding the patient's preference. A variation on this is **collaborative decision-making**. As proposed by Peisah et al. (2013), collaboration in this case is viewed as the physician informing the patient about the various treatment options that are available while simultaneously inviting the patient to describe his or her daily life, values, and goals, thus informing the healthcare team about areas of daily living that are meaningful to the patient. Collaborative decision-making goes a step beyond the shared decision-making model because it allows for more participants than only the patient and the physician. It can include family members, support system members, and advocates. In this case, the decision-making occurs as part of constructing a care plan, and collaboration occurs in every aspect of caregiving. Helping the patient to express what he or she views as being most important in life will enable the patient and help compensate for any limitations in ability to communicate.

Peisah et al. (2013) has proposed use of a model of supported decision-making that uses principles of collaboration while building on autonomy. It uses the acronym ASK ME:

1. **Assess** the patient's strengths and potential deficits. Deficits might include working memory, ability to weigh alternatives, ability to project consequences, or overall communication. Strengths could include having multiple supportive family members. Once the healthcare team is aware of the patient's strengths and weaknesses, it will be easier to change various aspects of the task so that the patient's ability to understand is maximized.
2. **Simplify** the task. A person is more likely to participate in decision-making for a simple decision than for a large, overarching decision. Avoid medical terms and use simplified language so that the information can be provided at the person's level of understanding.
3. **Know** the person. Determine what the person considers to be of most relevance in life and what their values are. Try to determine a past pattern of decision-making.
4. **Maximize** the ability to understand. Try to determine all factors that might complicate and slow the communication process so that they can be remedied. Provide as much time as possible and make the environment communication-friendly by providing optimal light, decreasing background noise, and providing privacy. Simplify information and make it as accessible as possible by increasing font size of type, reading information to the patient if needed, and providing illustrations if helpful. Pictorial representations of the choices can usually help the patient who is making a decision. Try to approach the patient at the time of day that is best for him or her rather than after the person has undergone a grueling treatment.
5. **Enable** the patient's participation in decision-making by providing a degree of support congruent to the complexity of the

decision and the potential consequences that could result from the decision.

DUTY TO WARN

If supportive decision-making proves to be ineffective and the patient's mental health continues to deteriorate, the nurse may experience an ethical dilemma based on conflict between the need to maintain confidentiality on the patient's history and a **duty to warn**. The concepts of duty to warn and **duty to protect** developed out of the **Tarasoff principle**, an offshoot of a 1974 legal case. The case initially began in 1968 when Prosenjit Poddar, a University of California, Berkeley student, developed an unreciprocated attraction to Tatiana Tarasoff. Mr. Poddar began to experience mental health issues during 1969 and sought counseling. During these sessions in August 1969, he revealed to his psychologist that he intended to kill Ms. Tarasoff. The psychologist notified university police of the situation and asked that they escort Mr. Poddar to a hospital for an involuntary mental health examination. Campus police detained and interviewed Mr. Poddar but then released him. In October 1969, Mr. Poddar arrived at Ms. Tarasoff's residence and killed her through a combination of shooting her with a pellet gun and stabbing her. He was subsequently charged with second-degree murder but was released after five years on the condition that he return to his home country of India. This led to Ms. Tarasoff's parents filing a lawsuit against the University of California, which resulted in the Tarasoff I decision. The ruling stated that mental health providers must warn potential victims of their danger ("duty to warn"). The case was retried in 1976, and the result was Tarasoff II. This ruling stated that clinicians have a duty to warn potential victims and that reasonable precautions must be taken to protect these third parties from the significant danger posed by patients such as Mr. Poddar ("duty to protect") (Gorshkalova & Munakomi, 2025).

The nurse who is experiencing an ethical dilemma based on a conflict between the need to maintain confidentiality of patient data and a duty to protect should consult the guidelines established by the American Psychiatric Association in 1987 regarding this. The guidelines state that for the clinician to have a duty to protect, four conditions must be present:

- The patient must express a clear threat of at least significantly injuring a reasonably identified victim, or
- The patient must voice threats of property destruction that can place others in danger,

- The patient must express intent, and
- The patient must possess the ability to execute the threat.

The guidelines indicate that clinicians must take "reasonable precautions" to protect third parties when such conditions are present. These precautions will consist of notifying the victims that have been identified by the patient, informing law enforcement personnel, and potentially hospitalizing the patient if necessary (Gorshkalova & Munakomi, 2025).

In summary, this chapter has discussed various ethical issues and challenges that can face the nurse who is working with a vulnerable patient population such as that of individuals experiencing mental illness. Another type of vulnerable patient group emerged in 2019 with the advent of the COVID-19 pandemic. The subsequent chapter will discuss ethical issues related to this recent phenomenon.

REFERENCES

Bernert, R. A., & Roberts, L. W. (2012). Ethics Commentary: Suicide Risk: Ethical considerations in the assessment and management of suicide risk. *FOCUS*, *10*(4), 467–472. https://doi.org/10.1176/appi.focus.10.4.467

Doyle, D., & Sollins, H. (2023). Decisional capacity—When and how to determine. *Caring for the Ages*, *24*(1), 16.

Gorshkalova, O., & Munakomi, S. (2025). Duty to warn. In *StatPearls* [Internet]. StatPearls Publishing. https://www.ncbi.nlm.nih.gov/books/NBK542236/

Hem, M. H., Gjerberg, E., Husum, T. L., & Pedersen, R. (2018). Ethical challenges when using coercion in mental healthcare: A systematic literature review. *Nursing Ethics*, *25*(1), 92–110. https://doi.org/10.1177/0969733016629770

National Institute of Mental Health. (n.d.). Suicide. Retrieved May 17, 2025, from https://www.nimh.nih.gov/health/statistics/suicide

Peisah, C., Sorinmade, O. A., Mitchell, L., & Hertogh, C. M. (2013). Decisional capacity: Toward an inclusionary approach. *International Psychogeriatrics*, *25*(10), 1571–1579. https://doi.org/10.1017/S1041610213001014.

NCLEX FORMAT REVIEW QUESTIONS

Match the area of determining decisional capacity with its description.

1. _____ understanding
2. _____ appreciation
3. _____ reasoning
4. _____ choice

a. Can the patient rationally evaluate the treatment alternatives as well as the diagnosis in terms of the ratio of risk to potential benefits, particularly in consideration of the impact on activities of daily living?

b. Can the patient understand the information related to the treatment plan and the overall diagnosis?

c. Can the patient clearly communicate a decision about his or her willingness or reluctance to participate in recommended treatments or tests?

d. Is the patient able to relate the information about the treatment plan and diagnosis to his or her own situation, particularly in terms of the potential benefits and harm?

Correct answers:

1. b
2. d
3. a
4. c

Arrange the stages of the model of supported decision-making in correct order.

5. a. _____ **Enable** the patient's participation in decision-making
   b. _____ **Know** the person
   c. _____ **Maximize** the ability to understand
   d. _____ **Assess** the patient's strengths and potential deficits
   e. _____ **Simplify** the task

Correct answer: d, e, b, c, a

6. Which ethical principle is viewed as the ability to self-govern?
   a. fidelity
   b. integrity
   c. autonomy
   d. veracity

Correct answer: c

7. Which ethical principle is viewed as providing fair treatment without evidence of prejudice?
   a. veracity
   b. justice

c. integrity
d. fidelity

Correct answer: b

8. Which ethical principle can best be described as being truthful with the patient?
   a. fidelity
   b. justice
   c. nonmaleficence
   d. veracity

Correct answer: d

9. Conditions that must be present for the clinician to have a duty to protect include: (select all that apply)
   a. the patient must express a clear threat of significantly injuring an identified victim
   b. the patient must possess the ability to execute the threat
   c. the patient must both voice and document threats of property destruction
   d. the patient must express intent

Correct answer: a, b, d

10. Reasonable precautions that should be used by clinicians to protect third parties include: (Select all that apply)
    a. potentially hospitalizing the patient if necessary
    b. informing law enforcement personnel
    c. notifying the victims that have been identified by the patient
    d. notifying the patient's family members as a safeguard

Correct answer: a, b, c

TEAM-BUILDING EXERCISE

Instructions: Divide students into teams of at least three people and preferably no more than five. Each person should have a role assigned in the exercise. One person will be the leader, one person will be the timekeeper, and one person will be the recorder. The **leader** will oversee helping the discussion progress so that the objectives of the exercise are accomplished. The **timekeeper** should intervene when necessary to keep the discussion focused on the topic of the exercise and should periodically remind team members of the amount of time remaining to complete the exercise. The **recorder** will be responsible for taking notes during the discussion that can be utilized when the exercise results are presented to the class. If additional team members are included in the group, one person can be assigned to assist with the notetaking and transcription process, and the additional person can assist the team leader in guiding the discussion and assist in preparing the final presentation of the results.

SCENARIO FOR TEAM-BUILDING EXERCISE

Sue is a 56-year-old female who has experienced symptoms of schizophrenia since her first psychotic break at the age of 19. She typically experiences both visual and auditory hallucinations and must be closely supervised to stay on her prescribed medication regimen. Sue's symptoms have been intensifying in recent years, and she is no longer a candidate to live in a group home in the community because of her occasional episodes of violence. She has moved back home with her 80-year-old mother. Sue's 50-year-old brother has been discussing the possibility of requesting a guardianship for her. Sue's mother is against this situation unless the mother can be named as guardian.

QUESTIONS

1. Discuss the ethical principles that will be applicable to Sue's situation if she becomes suicidal. Describe how each one could be individualized to her situation and how an ethical dilemma could result.

2. What type of process must be undertaken to determine whether Sue is considered to be competent?

3. Discuss the process of guardianship in Sue's case. In the role of nurse advocate for Sue, what would you consider to be most beneficial for her regarding guardianship?

4. Which areas will a face-to-face interview with Sue assess if capacity is being determined?

5. Compare and contrast shared decision-making, collaborative decision-making, and supportive decision-making. Do you think that any of these would be applicable to Sue's situation? Be able to support your answer.

6. Sue's condition continues to deteriorate. Which conditions must be present in order for the nurse to have a "duty to protect" in this case?

7. Sue threatens her brother and his family. What would be considered to be the "reasonable precautions" that should be implemented in this case?

CHAPTER 9

ETHICAL ISSUES PERTAINING TO THE PANDEMIC

CHAPTER OBJECTIVES

After studying this chapter, students will be able to:

- Discuss the American Nurses Association's ethical practice standards for nursing.
- Describe the influence of distributive justice on provision of care during a pandemic.
- Compare an egalitarian approach with a utilitarian approach to provision of care during a pandemic.
- Describe a nurse's duty to care.
- Discuss the reciprocity principle and the reciprocal responsibilities of hospitals.
- Compare duty to care with duty to promote equity and moral equality.
- Describe the crisis standard of care.
- Describe a framework for values at risk during a pandemic.

KEY TERMS

crisis standard of care
distributive justice
duty of care
duty to promote equity and moral equality
egalitarian approach
proportionality
reciprocity principle
utilitarian approach

The recent pandemic set the stage for nurses to experience ethical issues and dilemmas that most had never previously encountered.

The American Nurses Association's *Code of Ethics for Nurses With Interpretive Statements* (2015) provides the ethical practice standard for the nursing profession. The code indicates that the nurse's primary commitment must be to the patient, but also that the nurse owes the same duty to himself or herself as that provided to the patient. The obligations can easily conflict during a disaster such as a pandemic, when nurses must care for infectious patients under extreme duress, often without sufficient resources, and at increased risk to their own health. According to the American Nurses Association (ANA; n.d.), a disaster situation such as a pandemic may cause the nurse to be required to make a choice based on moral grounds in order to maintain professional integrity. Nurses may also struggle with the need to respond as a volunteer during a state of emergency if they belong to a vulnerable group, if they feel physically unsafe due to a lack of personal protective equipment, or if they are concerned about professional and ethical protection for providing nursing care during a disaster.

The American Nurses Association (n.d.) further notes that the nurse is responsible for having sufficient knowledge about state law regarding practicing during emergency situations such as a pandemic. According to the ANA, the nurse should research information regarding:

- State laws' mandates on the situations in which nurses must provide care,
- Protection for the nurse's license during crisis situations such as a pandemic, and
- Protection against lawsuits for negligence or malpractice for nurses who are practicing outside of their specialty areas in a disaster.

Sese et al. (2020) noted that the ethical framework in a public health crisis of this magnitude moves to promotion of public health through using resources with discretion so as to maximize lives saved. The rights of the individual patient by necessity must be minimized in order to most effectively utilize resources.

One of the main problems facing healthcare team members during the recent pandemic was the difficulty in providing sufficient medical resources, such as personal protective equipment, to promote public health. As rationing began to be implemented in some countries, the principles of **distributive justice** provided guidance on the correct way to distribute such resources. In light of a disaster such as a pandemic, an **egalitarian approach** to justice could be used to ensure that healthcare and medical resources are equally distributed among all patients and healthcare workers. Therefore, an ethically justified distribution of resources during the pandemic would have three goals:

- Efficient decision-making so that resources are dedicated to the individuals at greatest risk,
- Equity so that all patients are treated in a similar manner, and
- Prioritization so that resources are available to patients having the greatest need at any specific point in time.

In comparison, a **utilitarian approach** to the management of resources during the pandemic would have sought to maximize the total benefit for patients, which in this case would have meant extending life expectancy. This meant that using such an approach would have led to the distribution of supplies based on whether it would increase the number of patients recovering. Although under normal circumstances such an approach would be considered acceptable, given the time constraints faced by decision-makers during the pandemic, an egalitarian approach most often had to be implemented in order to maximize survival rates. This potentially led to an ethical dilemma and moral distress for healthcare team members as they struggled to decide which patients should be prioritized for treatment and how to distribute dwindling medical resources (Yuk-Chiu Yip, 2021).

Other ethical issues pertaining to the pandemic were documented by Wu and Kong (2023). These researchers noted that a significant ethical challenge for nurses during the pandemic was inaccurate emergency triage. Over-triage led to competition for resources for disease prevention, thus impacting distributive justice. In comparison, under-triage of patients led to limitations of individual patient autonomy.

The ethical principle of autonomy was the basis for another ethical dilemma for nurses that focused on the requirement of mandatory vaccination for some populations such as healthcare workers. Many nurses were conflicted between the duty to protect, beneficence, and nonmaleficence. Also, there was the question of whether the need to enforce personal autonomy included the right to potentially jeopardize the health of the public. In some cases, individual autonomy had to be limited to avoid exposing vulnerable populations to workers who had chosen to remain unvaccinated (Olick et al., 2021).

Another ethical issue unique to the pandemic arose out of the intensification of crowding in emergency departments. This also led to conflicts between individual patient interests and the interests of the public. In addition, an ethical challenge was presented by the inaccurate assessment of patient information during the pandemic via tele-triage, thus leading to the dilemma of inaccurate device feedback information and patient safety issues. Increasing reliance on devices for telephone triage was found to increase the probability of a privacy violation (Wu & Kong, 2023).

A different category of ethical dilemma developed for healthcare team members during the pandemic based on the duty of care as well as the reciprocity principle. The **duty of care** means that nurses and other team members were ethically required to act as advocates for patients, particularly while family members and support system members were unable to be present at the bedside due to isolation measures. This was occurring while staff members were also implementing safety measures and standard precautions and potentially endangering their own lives (Sahebi et al., 2020). In addition, the **reciprocity principle** states that hospitals have reciprocal responsibilities regarding staff, meaning that the organization needed to implement measures to support staff, such as:

- effective communication,
- interventions to control the spread of disease,
- efforts to motivate staff to carry out assigned duties,
- provision of adequate resources such as personal protective equipment,
- provision of training needed to generate a safe environment,
- provision of both psychological and medical care to staff affected by disease, and
- making staff a priority when vaccination became available.

An ethical dilemma would have resulted for healthcare staff members if they were providing patient care during the pandemic while the healthcare organization was struggling to provide the necessary infrastructure. Many hospitals were not able to meet all of the conditions considered to be reciprocal while the pandemic was at its height (Sahebi et al., 2020).

During public health crises such as the recent pandemic, the priorities of healthcare providers will change. Their obligations will compete with each other and create conflict for providers who are trained to focus on the individual patient. The two primary ethical obligations that will need to be balanced are:

- **duty to care**—focuses on the relief of suffering and a respect for the rights and preferences of the individual patient and
- **duty to promote equity and moral equality**—fairness is viewed as being relative to need when considering the distribution of risk and the benefit of care provision to public health.

As caregivers utilize ethical reasoning, they must consider what will ethically be of greatest benefit to the patient as well as being most feasible. This is considered to be the **crisis standard of care**, meaning that the limitations during a time of scarcity such as the pandemic are recognized. This type of ethical guidance is based on the duty to oversee resources according to transparency, consistency, **proportionality** (distribution according to need and the severity of the situation), and accountability (Sese et al., 2020).

In an effort to provide ethical guidance, the Pandemic Influenza Working Group at the University of Toronto Joint Centre for Bioethics developed a framework for values at risk during a pandemic based on a series of questions. See Box 9.1 for details.

BOX 9.1 (SESE ET AL., 2020)

Are restrictions on normal activities ethically justified?

At risk is individual liberty. All personal and professional practices must be reviewed on a regular basis and updated for the length of the pandemic to guarantee fairness of the application process.

How much more restrictive can measures ethically be for individuals and communities?

At risk are the values of justice and autonomy, with the primary obligation being that of protecting the public from harm. Restrictions will be required to be implemented by healthcare facilities in a public health crisis. Ethical reasoning for the restrictions should be the minimal amount necessary to protect both the public and individuals from either infection or transmission of the disease process.

Is it a HIPAA violation to report a diagnosis of the disease to public health officials?

At risk are the values of privacy and integrity, with the primary obligation being that of patients' health. In a situation such as a pandemic, the patient's right to privacy will be overridden in an effort to protect the public. The restrictions imposed will be the minimal needed to accomplish the goal while maintaining complete transparency with patients.

Who has the greatest right to receive personal protective equipment?

At risk is the value of needing to protect employees as well as the overarching community, with the overriding value being that of needing to provide care. Healthcare workers should be prioritized during the distribution of personal protective equipment since they have a duty to care for patients even when this places them at increased risk of illness.

How will public health officials and healthcare leaders decide how to distribute resources when a scarcity of supplies develops?

At risk is the value of providing each patient with what is required to meet his or her individual needs, with the overarching values being those of stewardship and utility of resources as well as transparency to patients. Although it is vital that medical equipment and treatment are distributed equitably and according to the benefit expected from such distribution, during a disaster such as a pandemic, parameters will shift to focus on triage so that patients who have the greatest expectation of recovery receive medical resources.

What should the public expect pertaining to updates on healthcare institutions making decisions?

At risk are time and resources being expended by the healthcare team, with the overriding value being the need to maintain transparency with patients. Although decisions should be made using as much transparency for patients as possible, the allocation of resources and possible change in procedures by healthcare workers will need to be based on a combination of values, principles, and supporting evidence.

Adapted from Denise Sese, Mahwish U. Ahmad, and Prabalini Rajendram, Selection from "Ethical Considerations During the COVID-19 Pandemic," *Cleveland Clinic Journal of Medicine*, vol. 92, no. 8, p. 3, https://www.ccjm.org/content/early/2020/06/01/ccjm.87a.ccc038. Copyright © 2025 by The Cleveland Clinic Foundation.

In summary, the unique ethical issues pertaining to the recent pandemic have been reviewed in light of their impact on future disastrous situations. Lessons learned from such a global state of emergency continue to unfold. It is the responsibility of nurses to glean as much knowledge as possible on this historical event to prevent future ethical dilemmas. The subsequent chapter will discuss future ethical dilemmas that could confront nurses in the 21st century and beyond.

REFERENCES

American Nurses Association. (n.d.). Nurses, ethics, and the response to the COVID-19 pandemic. Retrieved June 17, 2025, from https://www.nursingworld.org/globalassets/covid19/nurses-ethics-and-the-response-to-the-covid-19-pandemic_pdf-1.pdf

American Nurses Association. (2015). *Code of ethics for nurses with interpretive statements.* American Nurses Association.

Olick, R., Shaw, J., & Yang, T. (2021). Ethical issues in mandating COVID-19 vaccinations for health care personnel. *Mayo Clinic Proceedings, 96*(12), 2958–2962.

Sahebi, A., Moayedi, S., & Golitaleb, M. (2020). COVID-19 pandemic and the ethical challenges in patient care. *Journal of Medical Ethics and History of Medicine, 13*, 24. https://doi.org/10.18502/jmehm.v13i24.4955

Sese, D., Ahmad, M. U., & Rajendram, P. (2020). Ethical considerations during the COVID-19 pandemic. *Cleveland Clinic Journal of Medicine*. https://doi.org/10.3949/ccjm.87a.ccc038

Wu, L., & Kong, X. (2023). COVID-19 pandemic: Ethical issues and recommendations for emergency triage. *Frontiers Public Health, 11*, 1160769. https://doi.org/10.3389/fpubh.2023.1160769

Yuk-Chiu Yip, J. (2021). Healthcare resource allocation in the COVID-19 pandemic: Ethical considerations from the perspective of distributive justice within public health. *Public Health in Practice*, *2*(1), 100111. https://doi.org/10.1016/j.puhip.2021.100111

NCLEX FORMAT REVIEW QUESTIONS

1. According to the reciprocity principle, the reciprocal responsibilities of hospitals regarding staff include: (Select all that apply)

   a. _____ effective communication

   b. _____ interventions to control the spread of disease

   c. _____ provision of adequate staffing patterns

   d. _____ efforts to motivate staff to carry out assigned duties

   e. _____ provision of adequate resources such as personal protective equipment

   f. _____ provision of training needed to generate a safe environment

   g. _____ provision of both psychological and medical care to staff affected by disease

   h. _____ making staff a priority when vaccination is available

   Correct answer: a, b, d, e, f, g, h

2. The ethical obligation that focuses on the relief of suffering and a respect for the rights and preferences of the individual patient is known as:

   a. _____ duty to promote equity and moral equality

   b. _____ crisis standard of care

   c. _____ duty to care

   d. _____ proportionality

   Correct answer: c

3. The ethical obligation that views fairness as being relative to need when considering the distribution of risk and the benefit of care provision to public health is known as:

   a. ____ duty to promote equity and moral equality

   b. ____ crisis standard of care

   c. ____ duty to care

   d. ____ proportionality

Correct answer: a

4. When caregivers consider what will be ethically of greatest benefit to the patient as well as being most feasible, they are utilizing:

   a. ____ duty to care

   b. ____ consistency

   c. ____ crisis standard of care

   d. ____ proportionality

Correct answer: c

5. The crisis standard of care is a type of ethical guidance based on the duty to oversee resources according to: (Select all that apply)

   a. ____ transparency

   b. ____ consistency

   c. ____ severity

   d. ____ proportionality

   e. ____ accountability

Correct answer: a, b, d, e

6. According to the American Nurses Association, the nurse is responsible for having sufficient knowledge about state law regarding practicing during a pandemic. This means that the nurse should research information regarding: (Select all that apply)

   a. ____ State laws' mandates on the situations in which nurses must provide care

   b. ____ State laws' mandates regarding adequate staffing requirements

c. _____Protection for the nurse's license during crisis situations such as a pandemic

d. _____Protection against lawsuits for nurses practicing outside of their specialty areas

Correct answer: a, c, d

TEAM-BUILDING EXERCISE

Instructions: Divide students into teams of at least three people and preferably no more than five. Each person should have a role assigned in the exercise. One person will be the leader, one person will be the timekeeper, and one person will be the recorder. The **leader** will oversee helping the discussion progress so that the objectives of the exercise are accomplished. The **timekeeper** should intervene when necessary to keep the discussion focused on the topic of the exercise and should periodically remind team members of the amount of time remaining to complete the exercise. The **recorder** will be responsible for taking notes during the discussion that can be utilized when the exercise results are presented to the class. If additional team members are included in the group, one person can be assigned to assist with the notetaking and transcription process, and the additional person can assist the team leader in guiding the discussion and assist in preparing the final presentation of the results.

SCENARIO FOR TEAM-BUILDING EXERCISE

John is working as a nurse manager on a medical intensive care unit during a pandemic. The hospital is having difficulty in supplying employees with sufficient personal protective equipment. Many nurses have left their positions through retirement because of fear of jeopardizing the health of family members. John's unit is chronically understaffed; he is working an average of 60 hours per week. He has been losing about two employees a week lately. One of John's newest employees, a 22-year-old who just received her nurse's license, quit this morning. She tells him, "I can't risk taking this disease home to my husband and my baby!" John is very discouraged and for the first time in his career begins to consider the possibility of leaving bedside care and taking a position in academia.

QUESTIONS

1. Describe the American Nurses Association's views on the responsibilities of a nurse regarding knowledge about practicing during emergency situations such as a pandemic.

2. Discuss how use of an egalitarian approach to justice could assist John in his role as a nurse manager.

3. How will John and the other ICU nurses be influenced by the duty to care?

4. How will John and the other ICU nurses be influenced by the duty to promote equity and moral equality?

5. What are the reciprocal responsibilities of the hospital regarding John's staff members according to the reciprocity principle?

6. Describe how John will oversee the resources that are available to him according to:

   a. transparency

   b. consistency

c. proportionality

d. accountability

7. Use the framework for values at risk during a pandemic to analyze John's situation as nurse manager. Help him make crucial decisions regarding the intensive care unit, the staff, and his career.
   a. Are restrictions on normal activities ethically justified?
   b. How much more restrictive can measures ethically be for individuals and communities?
   c. Is it a HIPAA violation to report a diagnosis of the disease to public health officials?

d. Who has the greatest right to receive personal protective equipment?

e. How will public health officials and healthcare leaders decide how to distribute resources when a scarcity of supplies develops?

f. What should the public expect pertaining to updates on healthcare institutions making decisions?

CHAPTER 10

ETHICAL ISSUES PERTAINING TO NURSING IN THE FUTURE

CHAPTER OBJECTIVES

After studying this chapter, students will be able to:

- Discuss the use of algorithms in artificial intelligence.
- Describe how use of artificial intelligence can inadvertently perpetuate biases.
- Discuss external sources of bias in artificial intelligence.
- Describe specific strategies for mitigating bias and promoting health equity in artificial intelligence.
- Discuss the ethical principles that are essential to use of artificial intelligence.
- Discuss the use of facial recognition technology and its relationship to the Health Insurance Portability and Accountability Act (HIPAA).
- Discuss the importance of the Genetic Information Nondiscrimination Act (GINA) and its relationship to patients.
- Analyze the ethical issues that can pertain to genomics.
- Analyze the ethical issues pertaining to CRISPR technology.
- Discuss the concerns surrounding genome editing.

KEY TERMS

algorithm
Americans With Disabilities Act of 1990
artificial intelligence
bias
biodiversity
CRISPR technology
facial recognition technology
Genetic Information Nondiscrimination Act (GINA)

genetics
genome editing
genomics
health equity
Health Insurance Portability and Accountability Act (HIPAA)

The discussion thus far has focused on ethical issues and dilemmas that have plagued nurses in some cases since the advent of modern medicine. However, as healthcare moves farther into the 21st century, nurses must be prepared to face new ethical issues that will emerge from new medical breakthroughs and technological advances. A prime example of this is the use of **artificial intelligence** (AI) and robotics in healthcare. Although it holds out the promise of enhancing patient care through improved diagnostic processes and innovations, the use of AI includes its own set of ethical issues. For example, Elendu et al. (2023) noted that the use of AI generates large amounts of patient data that must be kept secure. Facilities will need to have policies and practices implemented for the collection, storage, and encryption of patient information. Rigby (2019) indicated that keeping patient photographic images would create ethical issues pertaining to autonomy because of facial recognition technology that could threaten the ability to obtain proper informed consent.

Each healthcare institution will need to adhere to data security standards such as those included in the Health Insurance Portability and Accountability Act. Security protocols will have to be updated frequently to adapt to new cybersecurity threats. In addition, the algorithms used in AI have been found to inadvertently perpetuate biases in healthcare data that can lead to diagnostic disparities and potential errors in treatment. Each facility will need to have algorithms that will eliminate bias in making healthcare decisions (Elendu et al., 2023).

The potential for artificial intelligence to transform healthcare from its current iteration is almost unlimited. However, for this to occur, both health equity and ethical practice must be observed. **Health equity** in this case refers to the fair and just distribution of health technology and its benefits. This means that all individuals will have access to the same quality of healthcare services regardless of race, gender, ethnicity, geographic locale, or socioeconomic status. For AI to be most transformative, it must be able to narrow existing health disparities. This can only occur through elimination of **bias**. Bias in artificial intelligence means that the AI system has been designed so that the system makes unfair decisions that can result from lack of research diversity. AI models are usually trained on currently available data, which may not sufficiently represent all racial and ethnic minority groups, many of which are medically underserved. Although AI bias usually involves **algorithms**, which are the set of instructions provided to the computer to complete a task, external sources of bias can also exist (Dankwa-Mullan, 2024). These include the following:[1]

- Experience and expertise—this bias is introduced by the various levels of expertise among the individuals who develop an AI system. For example, if all developers are not consistently familiar with AI tools, there will be differences in how the tools are implemented and interpreted. Also, inadequate expertise can lead to incorrect labeling of data as well as choosing models that don't generalize well when applied to diverse populations.
- Exclusion—this bias is introduced when certain groups are systematically left out of data collection and analysis. This will result in an AI system that doesn't accurately represent the entire population. If an AI tool is developed without considering populations that have been marginalized either socially or economically, the tool won't address barriers faced by specific groups when attempting to access healthcare.
- Environment—this bias develops from the socio-environmental conditions under which the data are collected and utilized. This bias can include the social determinants of health, such as income, education, and living conditions, as well as the physical environment, both geographic locale and urban or rural environment. When environmental factors are incorporated appropriately into an AI model, it will more effectively mitigate health disparities.
- Empathy—this type of bias refers to the difficulty encountered when attempting to incorporate human experiences into an AI system. The system may not be able to accurately utilize qualitative data or consider patient preferences and values.
- Evidence—this type of bias pertains to the process by which scientific evidence is generated, disseminated into the scientific community, and ultimately becomes the basis for practice. The method of funding research can be problematic since funding priorities may not meet the needs of all populations. The development of clinical guidelines from evidence can produce bias if patient diversity is not considered (Dankwa-Mullan, 2024).

---

1. Adapted from Irene Dankwa-Mullan/Centers for Disease Control and Prevention (CDC), Selections from "Health Equity and Ethical Considerations in Using Artificial Intelligence in Public Health and Medicine," *Preventing Chronic Disease*, vol. 21, no. 64, pp. 3–4, https://www.cdc.gov/pcd/issues/2024/24_0245.htm, U.S. Department of Health and Human Services, 2024.

There are methods for mitigating bias and promoting health equity in AI. This can occur through collection of data from diverse populations, developing AI with explainable outcomes to ensure accountability, monitoring for biased outcomes, and adjusting algorithms to make certain they remain equitable. Specific strategies include the following:

- Experience and expertise bias—develop teams with diverse expertise; provide ongoing training for healthcare team members to ensure that they have proficiency in AI tool interpretation. Develop standardized protocols for data collection and algorithm development to decrease the possibility of variability.
- Exclusion bias—ensure that datasets include diverse demographic groups. Conduct regularly scheduled audits of AI systems to identify evidence of population exclusion. Design AI tools that are accessible to marginalized groups.
- Environment bias—ensure that AI models include social determinants of health. This should allow for a more holistic understanding of AI health outcomes. Use geospatial analysis to include environmental factors such as air quality and water access in health data. Adapt AI models so that they account for regional variations in the social and environmental factors that can influence health.
- Empathy bias—combine quantitative data with qualitative data from patient interviews to provide a more complete picture of a patient's health. Include patients in the design of AI systems to verify that the models reflect patient preferences, values, and experiences. Include patient representatives on ethical review boards to align AI tools with patient needs and ethical standards.
- Evidence bias—diversify funding sources to ensure that research is supported that addresses the health needs of marginalized groups. Encourage transparency in reporting both positive and negative research findings. Develop inclusive clinical guidelines to build an evidence base that is free of bias and comprehensive.

Using these strategies will show that, although bias in AI will challenge health equity, incorporating ethical principles can allow an opportunity to enhance healthcare for multiple patient populations. If equity is made a priority in AI design, healthcare team members can use these tools to improve health outcomes and also generate improvement across a diverse population (Dankwa-Mullan, 2024).

TABLE 10.1 EXTERNAL SOURCES OF BIAS

	Experience & Expertise	Exclusion	Environment	Empathy	Evidence
Description	introduced by various levels of expertise among individuals who develop an AI system	introduced when certain groups are systematically left out of data collection and analysis	develops from the socio-environmental conditions under which the data are collected and utilized	refers to the difficulty encountered when attempting to incorporate human experiences into an AI system	pertains to process by which scientific evidence is generated, disseminated into scientific community, and ultimately becomes basis for practice
Example	if all developers are not consistently familiar with AI tools, there will be differences in how tools are implemented and interpreted	if an AI tool is developed without considering populations that have been marginalized either socially or economically, the tool won't address barriers faced by specific groups when attempting to access healthcare	can include social determinants of health (income, education, living conditions, & physical environment, both geographic locale and urban or rural environment); if environmental factors are incorporated into an AI model, it will more effectively mitigate health disparities	system may not be able to accurately utilize qualitative data or consider patient preferences and values	method of funding research can be problematic since funding priorities may not meet the needs of all populations; development of clinical guidelines from evidence can produce bias if patient diversity is not considered
Strategies	develop teams with diverse expertise; provide ongoing training for team members to ensure that they have proficiency in AI tool interpretation; develop standardized protocols for data collection and algorithm development to decrease possibility of variability	ensure that datasets include diverse demographic groups; conduct regularly scheduled audits of AI systems to identify evidence of population exclusion; design AI tools that are accessible to marginalized groups	for a more holistic understanding of AI health outcomes; use geospatial analysis to include environmental factors such as air quality and water access into health data; adapt AI models so that they account for regional variations in social & environmental factors that can influence health	combine quantitative & qualitative data from patient interviews to complete picture of patient's health; include patients in the design of AI systems to verify that models reflect patient preferences, values, and experiences; include patient representatives on ethical review boards to align AI tools with patient needs and ethical standards	diversify funding sources to ensure that research is supported that addresses health needs of marginalized groups; encourage transparency in reporting both positive and negative research findings; develop inclusive clinical guidelines to build an evidence base that is free of bias and comprehensive

Adapted from Irene Dankwa-Mullan/Centers for Disease Control and Prevention (CDC), Selections from "Health Equity and Ethical Considerations in Using Artificial Intelligence in Public Health and Medicine," *Preventing Chronic Disease*, vol. 21, no. 64, pp. 3–4, https://www.cdc.gov/pcd/issues/2024/24_0245.htm, U.S. Department of Health and Human Services, 2024.

Once the decision is made by a healthcare facility to utilize artificial intelligence, the facility must also decide on the incorporation of various ethical frameworks that will guide clinical practice as well as the development of technology. These ethical frameworks must include various ethical principles pertaining to the use of AI in a healthcare arena. These ethical principles include: beneficence and nonmaleficence to make certain that use of AI will only be beneficial to patients and won't cause harm through either error or bias; maintenance of patient autonomy through transparency and obtaining the needed consents in interactions utilizing AI; and fairness and justice to verify that tools energized by AI don't worsen inequalities but instead provide increased access to services for patients. Use of artificial intelligence will necessitate the use of scrupulous security measures due to the vast amount of patient personal data that will be processed. Healthcare facilities should incorporate consent forms that include giving permission for patient images to be utilized and also that take into consideration patients who may speak English as a second language. Finally, facilities that incorporate use of AI must develop guidelines that require vigilant human oversight of decisions that are based on AI information. This will help ensure that AI sharpens rather than replaces human judgment (Dankwa-Mullan, 2024).

New issues regarding privacy and confidentiality have arisen pertaining to **facial recognition technology**. This type of technology uses software to map facial characteristics; this information will then be stored in the form of a face template. Algorithms will be applied to a database to compare facial images and identify patterns that can be used in diagnosing genetic disorders or providing indicators of the patient's health status. This means that informed consent will need to be obtained for the collection and storage of patients' images as well as the purposes for which the images are being analyzed by facial recognition technology systems. Patients may not be aware that their images can be used to generate additional clinical information. It is uncertain whether such information can be completely deidentified, and patients will need to be informed regarding this risk (Martinez-Martin, 2019).

Facial templates are classified as biometric data and as such contain information that can be used to potentially identify patients. The **Health Insurance Portability and Accountability Act (HIPAA)** addresses the use of patients' health records as well as personal health information and includes privacy protection for information that is considered personally identifiable, such as biometric data. Be aware that some statutes that will protect a patient's health information may not be applicable to use of facial recognition technology. For example, the **Genetic Information Nondiscrimination Act (GINA)**, which was signed into law in 2008, does not apply to facial recognition technology since it does not fit the statute's definition of either genetic testing or genetic information (Martinez-Martin, 2019). This statute protects against genetic discrimination in an employment setting or in obtaining and maintaining health insurance. It also ensures the privacy of individual and family genetic information (American Society of Human Genetics, n.d.). In addition, the **Americans With Disabilities Act of 1990**, although useful in protecting people with disabilities from discrimination in an academic or employment setting, for example, would probably not apply to facial recognition technology being used for the purpose of diagnosis (Martinez-Martin, 2019).

Additional ethical concerns come into consideration regarding the long-term impact of facial recognition technology. If use of such diagnostic software progresses to the point of replacing a physician's judgment, ethical and legal concerns will become paramount concerning where liability will lie. In addition, if such technology is utilized to monitor compliance with treatment regimens or assist in surveillance of patients, the patient-physician trust relationship will be undermined. Therefore, the specific benefits of facial recognition technology with identified populations of patients, as well as the responsibilities that come with its usage, must be weighed carefully (Martinez-Martin, 2019).

As AI and robotics continue to be integrated into healthcare, there will be new challenges for healthcare team members. For example, geographic disparities in healthcare may be inadvertently created as vulnerable populations are excluded because of inadequate access to technology such as telemedicine. In addition, there is a possibility of clinicians becoming dependent on use of AI at the risk of forgoing use of clinical judgment and patient assessment. It will be crucial for clinicians to verify that AI is being implemented to ensure that health disparities are changing positively and that patients in every demographic will benefit (Elendu et al., 2023).

Other ethical issues that are already in existence but will intensify in the future relate to genetics and genomics. **Genetics** refers to the study of individual genes associated with specific gene disorders that are often rare in the general population.

In contrast, **genomics** refers to the study of the entire human genome as well as influencing variables that may be personal, environmental, psychosocial, or cultural. The use of genomic information carries with it the possibility of discrimination against the person involved as well as his or her family members. An example of such intensifying ethical issues involves **CRISPR technology**, a gene-editing tool that allows scientists to target and modify DNA sequences within living cells. One significant ethical concern involves the safety of CRISPR technology, since it is known to result in both intended and unintended effects. These effects have the potential to harm the health of an organism that has been genetically edited as well as that of future generations. Another concern is that CRISPR technology could threaten **biodiversity**.

Biodiversity is both the presence of a wide variety of species and also genetic diversity within one species. The biodiversity of species is essential to the overall health of an ecosystem. **Genome editing** could increase the resilience of some endangered plant species, thus allowing their populations to rebound. The concern is that CRISPR-based tools could promote monoculture farming practices that can threaten biodiversity. In addition, cutting-edge, expensive technology such as CRISPR can potentially widen the gap between wealthy and struggling countries. Currently, CRISPR technology is being evaluated for its ability to treat diseases in cells that would not be passed down genetically. However, if it is used to create changes in sperm, eggs, or embryos that would be passed throughout a family, potentially the technology would only be available to the very wealthiest members of a society, thus potentially widening disparities in both the overall health of a nation and its economic striations. As CRISPR technology is increasingly used to engineer an approach to the human genome, concerns have been raised that it is being utilized as a form of eugenics to eliminate individuals considered to be disabled (Henderson et al., 2024).

In summary, the nurse who practices in years to come will face ethical challenges pertaining to many areas, such as genetics and genomics, but certainly some of the most significant challenges will pertain to use of artificial intelligence. The potential for patient–healthcare team member interactions to become greatly dehumanized is significant if monitoring does not occur. However, the same potential exists for use of AI in the hands of professionals who are trained in ethical principles and practices to make huge inroads in progress toward the eradication of longstanding fatal diseases. It will be up to the 21st-century nurse to recognize the need to provide consistent monitoring as AI tools become ever more sophisticated.

REFERENCES

American Society of Human Genetics. (n.d.). The Genetic Information Discrimination Act (GINA). Retrieved July 10, 2025, from https://www.ashg.org/advocacy/gina/

Dankwa-Mullan, I. (2024). Health equity and ethical considerations in using artificial intelligence in public health and medicine. *Preventing Chronic Disease, 21*, 240245. http://dx.doi.org/10.5888/pcd21.240245

Elendu, C., Amaechi, D. C., Elendu, T. C., Jingwa, K. A., Okoye, O. K., John Okah, M., Ladele, J. A., Farah, A. H., & Alimi, H. A. (2023). Ethical implications of AI and robotics in healthcare: A review. *Medicine (Baltimore), 102*(50), e36671. https://doi.org/10.1097/MD.0000000000036671

Henderson, H. R., Ramit, G., Tolpa, T., Murdock, A. G., & Halpern, J. (2024) CRISPR & ethics. In Hochstrasser et al. (Eds.) *CRISPRpedia*. Innovative Genomics Institute, University of California, Berkeley. https://doi.org/10.60640/G2H59Q

Martinez-Martin, N. (2019). What are important ethical implications of using facial recognition technology in health care? *AMA Journal of Ethics, 21*(2), E180–187. https://doi.org/10.1001/amajethics.2019.180

Rigby, M. (2019). Ethical dimensions of using artificial intelligence in health care. *AMA Journal of Ethics, 21*(2), E121–124. https://doi.org/10.1001/amajethics.2019.121

NCLEX FORMAT REVIEW QUESTIONS

Match the external source of bias in artificial intelligence with the correct description.

a. experience and expertise
b. exclusion
c. environment
d. empathy
e. evidence

1. _____ refers to the difficulty encountered when attempting to incorporate human experiences into an AI system
2. _____ introduced when certain groups are systematically left out of data collection and analysis
3. _____ introduced by the various levels of expertise among the individuals who develop an AI system
4. _____ can develop if an AI tool is developed without considering populations that have been marginalized either socially or economically
5. _____ the tool won't address barriers faced by specific groups when attempting to access healthcare
6. _____ pertains to the process by which scientific evidence is generated, disseminated into the scientific community, and ultimately becomes the basis for practice

7. ____ AI tool is developed without considering populations that have been marginalized either socially or economically

Correct answers:

1. d	3. a	5. e	7. b
2. b	4. b	6. c	

Match the strategy for mitigating bias and promoting health equity in artificial intelligence with the appropriate type of bias.

a. experience and expertise
b. exclusion
c. environment
d. empathy
e. evidence

1. ____ ensure that datasets include diverse demographic groups
2. ____ combine quantitative data with qualitative data from patient interviews to provide a more complete picture of a patient's health
3. ____ include patient representatives on ethical review boards to align AI tools with patient needs and ethical standards
4. ____ conduct regularly scheduled audits of AI systems to identify evidence of population exclusion
5. ____ provide ongoing training for healthcare team members to ensure that they have proficiency in AI tool
6. ____ include patients in the design of AI systems to verify that the models reflect patient preferences, values, and experiences
7. ____ encourage transparency in reporting both positive and negative research findings
8. ____ design AI tools that are accessible to marginalized groups
9. ____ diversify funding sources to ensure that research is supported that addresses the health needs of marginalized groups
10. ____ develop standardized protocols for data collection and algorithm development to decrease the possibility of variability
11. ____ develop inclusive clinical guidelines to build an evidence base that is free of bias and comprehensive
12. ____ develop teams with diverse expertise

13. _____ adapt AI models so that they account for regional variations in the social and environmental factors that can influence health
14. _____ encourage transparency in reporting both positive and negative research findings
15. _____ ensure that AI models include social determinants of health
16. _____ use geospatial analysis to include environmental factors such as air quality and water access into health data
17. _____ system may not be able to accurately utilize qualitative data or consider patient preferences and values

Correct answers:

1. b	6. d	11. e	16. c
2. d	7. e	12. a	17. d
3. d	8. b	13. c	
4. b	9. e	14. e	
5. a	10. a	15. c	

TEAM-BUILDING EXERCISE

Instructions: Divide students into teams of at least three people and preferably no more than five. Each person should have a role assigned in the exercise. One person will be the leader, one person will be the timekeeper, and one person will be the recorder. The **leader** will oversee helping the discussion progress so that the objectives of the exercise are accomplished. The **timekeeper** should intervene when necessary to keep the discussion focused on the topic of the exercise and should periodically remind team members of the amount of time remaining to complete the exercise. The **recorder** will be responsible for taking notes during the discussion that can be utilized when the exercise results are presented to the class. If additional team members are included in the group, one person can be assigned to assist with the note-taking and transcription process, and the additional person can assist the team leader in guiding the discussion and assist in preparing the final presentation of the results.

SCENARIO FOR TEAM-BUILDING EXERCISE

The administration at Mercy Medical Center submitted a proposal last year to incorporate artificial intelligence in the form of facial recognition technology into the surgical area. The hospital was able to attract a new group of physicians who are trained to use the most cutting-edge surgical techniques. After using the technology for six months, it became obvious that it was biased against specific minority groups. If this is not corrected, the project will have to be discontinued and the hospital will lose millions of dollars in revenue annually. The surgical group is already threatening to affiliate with a different healthcare facility.

QUESTIONS

1. Discuss the policies and practices that the facility will need to develop and implement for the collection, storage, and encryption of patient information related to facial recognition technology.

2. Analyze the ethical issues that can exist pertaining to facial recognition technology.

3. Analyze the various sources of bias that could exist with facial recognition technology.

4. Discuss methods of mitigating bias and promoting health equity in the use of artificial intelligence, especially facial recognition technology.

5. Discuss the ethical principles that will be most applicable to using facial recognition technology.

6. Describe the issues regarding privacy and confidentiality that pertain to using facial recognition technology.

7. a. Discuss the relationship of the Health Insurance Portability and Accountability Act (HIPAA) to using facial recognition technology. If it is not applicable, explain why.

   b. Discuss the relationship of the Genetic Information Nondiscrimination Act (GINA) to using facial recognition technology. If it is not applicable, explain why.

   c. Discuss the relationship of the Americans With Disabilities Act of 1990 to using facial recognition technology. If it is not applicable, explain why.

INDEX

D

E

F

G

H

Q

R

S

T

U

V

W

www.ingramcontent.com/pod-product-compliance
Ingram Content Group UK Ltd.
Pitfield, Milton Keynes, MK11 3LW, UK
UKHW052002041026
15590UKWH00008B/2095